KU-692-756

Contents

Introduction to Reprinted Edition   1

Foreword to Reprinted Edition McFarlane of Llandaff   3

List of Tables   5

Acknowledgements   7

Preface   8

    Introduction

    A Study of Interpersonal Relationships in General
    Wards   10
    Summary of Conclusions   11

Part I

  1. *Problems, Hypotheses, Questions to be Answered,
      Aims and Method of Study*   12
    The Problem   12
    Two Hypotheses   12
    Questions   12
    Aims   12
    Method of Study   13

  2. *Developing à Tool for Assessing the Popularity and
      Unpopularity of Patients*   14
    Introduction   14
    A Rating Scale for Measuring Popularity   14
    A Ranking Scale for Measuring Popularity   16

  3. *Testing Factors that Might Account for Unpopularity*   18
    Results   19
      1. Use of popularity rating scales   19
      2. Use of popularity ranking scales   19
      3. The combined rating, ranking and comparative
          study wards   19
    Diagnosis   25
    Summary   25

4. *Nurses' Attitudes Towards Patients*   26
    Results   26
    Summary   27

5. *Exploring the Nurses' View of the Patients' Role*   28
    Introduction   28
    Development of the Role Definition Tool   29
    Results   30
    Summary of Part I   30

Part II

6. *Comparative Analysis Defined*   31

7. *Aims and Method of Comparison for this Study*   33
    Methods   33
        1. Non-participant selective observation   33
        2. Data collection from nurses and patients   34
        3. Assessment of popular and unpopular patients   34
        4. Semi-structured interviews with the nurses   34

8. *The Choice of Wards*   36

9. *Portraits of the Wards*   37
    Ash Ward   37
    Elm Ward   39
    Fir Ward   41
    Oak Ward   43

10. *Four Wards Compared*   45
    Observations of the patients' role in the wards   45
    Behaviour of popular patients   45
    Behaviour of least popular patients   46
    Attitudes expressed by the nurses about patients
    they most enjoyed caring for   49
    Attitudes expressed by the nurses about patients
    they least enjoyed caring for   50
    Use of sanctions   52
    Observations of nurse/patient interaction in the wards   53
    Patterns of interaction   53

Joking, teasing and banter   56
Nurses' attitudes to interaction with patients   58
Patients' attitudes to interaction with nurses   59
Summary of Part II   60

Part III

11. *Notes on the Theoretical Background to the
    Concept of Small Groups, Group Norms and Role*   62

    Groups   63
    Norms   63
    Role   64

12. *Likes and Dislikes in Group Situations*   66

13. *Abstracts from the Literature on Popular and
    Unpopular Patients*   69

Appendices

    1. Tables showing Factors found to have no Significant
       Influence on the Popularity of Patients   73

    2. Comments made by Nurses about Patients they
       Most and Least Enjoyed Caring For   77

    3. The Role Study   80
       (a) Results of Using Role Definition Tool   80
       (b) Results of 12 Item Questionnaire   82

    4. Data Collecting Schedules   83
       1. Rating Chart   83
       2. Classification of Patients   84
       3. Nursing Staff Questionnaire   86
       4. List of Statements about Patients   87

Bibliography   89

Introduction to Reprinted Edition

More than ten years have passed since *The Unpopular Patient* was first published. The fact that there is still a call for it that results in this reprinted edition has both positive and negative aspects. On the good side, it is an encouraging fact that the nursing profession is taking notice of research findings and both libraries and individuals are prepared to buy and find shelf space for, what is now, a greatly increased number of published reports. This is also evidenced by the large numbers of references to nursing research that are cited in many published articles and text books. The less good aspect about this reprinting is that there are indications that the findings of the study are still relevant.

When the study was undertaken in the late 1960s, there was very little factual information available about the nature of nurse–patient interaction and the extent to which patients' emotional needs were considered or catered for. With its original publication *The Unpopular Patient* received a very hostile reception from the nursing profession. In the time that has elapsed since then, other workers have studied relationships and communications between nurses and patients, and on the whole these studies show that there is still room for improved practice in these areas. What is encouraging now is that there seems to be much more questioning among nurses as to how improvement might be achieved.

As this publication is an account of a research study, it is reprinted in its original form. Readers who are interested in updated references to subsequent studies and their findings in the area of nursing relationships and communication skills, are referred to such books as:
Research for Nursing, J. MacCleod Clark and L. Hockey (H.M. & M. Publishers, Aylesbury, 1979); *Communication in Nursing Care*, edited by W. Bridge and J. MacCleod Clark (H.M. & M. Publishers, Aylesbury, 1981); and *Social Skills for Nursing Practice*, P. French (Croom Helm Publishers, London, 1983).

On a personal note I should like to refer readers to the literature abstracts in Chapter 13 and suggest, as some of these writers do, that by being kind, attentive and nice to people when they are being 'nasty' you are much more likely to improve their behaviour than by being curt, cross and ignoring them. If this study helps you to identify an unpopular patient or client in your care, perhaps you could try using the 'being nice' prescription and evaluate the outcome as a personal 'experiment'.

Felicity Stockwell

1

Foreword to Reprinted Edition

It is particularly useful that *The Unpopular Patient* should be reprinted because it is still in demand for its relevance to nursing practice and research ·methodology. It was one of a group of studies of nursing practice of which I was privileged to be the first co-ordinator, carried out over ten years ago at the Royal College of Nursing. The principal aim of the project (which owed its conception to Marjorie Simpson and its funding to the Department of Health and Social Security) was to develop techniques of measuring the quality of nursing care. This aim was not achieved because of the complexity of the subject and of the sophisticated research it necessitated. Nonetheless, the studies individually contributed insights into the nature of the quality of nursing care and pioneered research into nursing practice in the United Kingdom.

The Unpopular Patient in particular drew dramatic attention to the inadequacies of nurse–patient interaction. Writing the Preface in 1972 I said 'Few nurses will read this report with equanimity' and I have kept press cuttings which recall the hostility with which the report was received. Its findings are now, however, corroborated by a number of subsequent studies of communication in nursing which demonstrate continuing inadequacies in nursing practice and underline the relevance of the findings of this study today. The importance of nurses evaluating their own practice if they are to be accountable is gaining ground. From this study we find that patients do not receive individualised and holistic care nor are nurses skilful in interpersonal relationships. Despite changes in the curriculum of nursing education this has not altered. The implications are that there is a need for radical changes in practice, in the methods of education used for learning communication skills and in the managerial climate in which nurses relate to patients.

The Unpopular Patient pioneered new ground in research design and method. The group of studies in 'The Study of Nursing Care' Project were carried out by nurses at a time when few nurses in this country had any knowledge or experience of research methods; a programme of education in methodology was therefore part of the researcher's preparation. The studies were pioneering and learning experiences. In the light of professional progress in the intervening fifteen years some of the studies could well be criticised, and the generalisability of some of the findings can be questioned.

The Unpopular Patient, however, was a historical landmark in research design. First, it used both quantitative and qualitative approaches to the study of the same problem and so demonstrated the strength of

3

'triangulation' of methods (the process of using different methods to study the subject). Secondly, it was the first nursing research study in the UK to make use of the constant comparative method described by Glaser and Strauss (1968). The method has been more widely used in recent years, but it is eminently suitable to a young discipline needing to identify the phenomena and concepts in its field as a first stage of theory development. *The Unpopular Patient* served to identify categories of behaviour nurses use towards unpopular patients. Thus both in its implications for clinical practice and research, *The Unpopular Patient* continues to have relevance to students and practitioners of nursing and to educators, managers and researchers alike.

McFarlane of Llandaff

List of Tables

Table 1 Range of rating scores. Allocation Scores and Average Allocation Scores 15

Table 2 Percentage ranking scores allocated by the nurses to the most and least popular patients in each ward 17

Table 3 Previous hospitalization of the most and least popular patient 19

Table 4 Classification of patients by popularity 20

Table 5 Classification of patients by popularity of U.K. and foreign patients 20

Table 6 Classification of patients by popularity and country of origin 21

Table 7 Classification of patients by popularity and length of present stay in hospital 22

Table 8 Classification of patients by popularity and length of previous stay in hospital 23

Table 9 Classification of patients by popularity and defect 24

Table 10 Distribution of reasons given by two groups of different nurses for enjoying or not enjoying looking after patients 27

Table 11 Classification of patients by popularity and age 73

Table 12 Classification of patients by popularity and religious affiliation 74

Table 13 Classification of patients by popularity and social class 75

Table 14 Classification of patients by popularity and type of accommodation prior to present admission 76

Acknowledgements

I should like to express my gratitude to the Department of Health and Social Security and the Royal College of Nursing for giving me the opportunity, the finance and the tuition that made it possible for me to carry out this study.

For their help and supervision my thanks go to Miss H. M. Simpson, Nursing Officer (Research), D.O.H.S.S.; Miss J. K. McFarlane, Project Leader; Professor J. Woodward, Imperial College of Science and Technology, and the other members of the Steering Committee: Dr. J. A. D. Anderson, Miss M. F. Carpenter, Miss J. Cooper, and Dr. M. Scott Wright.

I am indebted to the nursing staff and patients in the wards in which the study was carrried out, and I am particularly grateful for the tolerance, help and interest extended to me by the ward sisters who were involved.

I owe especial thanks to Miss M. West for editing the study, to Mrs. U. Inman for her assistance, and to Mrs. J. Penney who typed the manuscript.

Lastly I should like to thank my husband and my colleagues on the project for their unfailing encouragement and support.

Preface

This study is one of a group undertaken as part of the research project "The Study of Nursing Care", sponsored by the Department of Health and Social Security, and administered by the Royal College of Nursing and National Council of Nurses of the United Kingdom.

The main objective of the project is to develop techniques for measuring the quality of nursing care. An account of the first two years of the project and its approach to measuring quality have been outlined in "The Proper Study of the Nurse" (McFarlane, Rcn. 1971). Nurses appointed to work with the project as research assistants selected an aspect of nursing care and studied it in depth. From these studies factors affecting the quality of care in a number of areas have emerged. The project has now entered a new phase in which measures of the quality of care developed for these individual aspects of nursing will be refined and built into an overall scale of quality.

The individual studies in isolation, therefore, do not achieve the main objective of the Project and were not designed to stand in isolation. They all, however, contribute factual information about the practice of nursing and their discussion by groups of nurses in hospitals or units could stimulate improvement in nursing care. It is for this reason that the individual studies are being published.

The Unpopular Patient is a study of interpersonal relationships between nurses and patients in general hospital wards. It deals with an aspect of nursing which pervades the whole of nursing function. It shows with clarity that nursing is not just a series of techniques or procedures, but concerns the care of persons. In this care the personality of the patient and the personality of the nurse interact. This report shows how that interaction may affect the quality of nursing care given.

Few nurses will read this report with equanimity. It should stimulate us to make greater efforts in the training of nurses so that emotional care of the patient is appreciated as a part of total patient care. It should help us to recognize that the study of behavioural sciences by nurses should be directed to an understanding of ourselves and our own human reactions to people as much as to an understanding of the patient. Leaders of professional teams such as ward sisters will recognize their part in creating a climate in which the human relations aspect of nursing will be recognized and maintained at a high standard.

TO JACK

INTRODUCTION

A Study of Interpersonal Relationships in General Wards

The original impetus for this study came from an interest in the care given to patients classified as "difficult" by the nursing staff, and from a need to know more about the problems presented by such patients in order to help nurses understand and care for them.

The requirements of the project, of which this study forms part, were to devise some means of assessing the quality of nursing care in general wards.

It was hoped to combine these two facets by exploring the nature of popularity and unpopularity of patients with nursing staff and determining whether there was any measurable difference in the quality of nursing care they received.

The study has devised means of identifying popular and unpopular patients, explored possible reasons for patients being thus classified and examined the nurses' attitudes and behaviour towards them.

A quantitative approach was originally formulated and carried out but it was eventually felt that more information about interactions in the ward situation was needed and therefore a qualitative "comparative analysis" was carried out to lay the foundations for more realistic measurements of nursing care in this area.

Summary of Conclusions

The chief aim of this study was to determine whether there were some patients whom the nursing team enjoyed caring for more than others and, if this proved to be so, to ascertain whether there was any measurable difference in the nursing care afforded to the most and least popular patients.

The first part of the work shows that it is possible for nurses to identify both popular and unpopular patients by means of the rating and ranking scales developed in the study. Of these, the ranking scale proved to be the more effective tool.

Reasons for patients' unpopularity were mostly related to personality factors and physical defects such as deafness but patients of foreign nationality and those whose present stay in hospital was longer than three months also proved to be significantly more unpopular than others.

In an attempt to gain more information about what might influence the nurses' enjoyment or lack of enjoyment in caring for particular patients, an attempt was made to define the nurses' view of the patient's role in the ward. In the process of a *comparative study* in four wards this was related to the patients the nurses stated they most enjoyed and least enjoyed caring for and to any variations in the amount and type of interaction that they had with them.

A quantitative evaluation of nurse/patient interaction was not attempted, but there were some observable differences in the ways in which nurses interacted with the most and the least popular patients.

In contrast with the findings of Viguers, R. T. (1959) this second part of the study showed that least attention was given to those mid-group bedfast patients who were neither particularly popular nor unpopular with the nursing staff. This finding was not anticipated.

On the whole, nurses felt that the carrying out of nursing tasks provided adequate opportunity for interaction with patients while the patients expressed in varying degree that they did not have enough contact with, or information from, the nurses. Both nurses and patients felt, however, that stopping just for conversation was not part of the nursing task.

PART I

CHAPTER 1

Problems, Hypotheses, Questions to be Answered, Aims and Method of Study

The Problem

The basic problem underlying this study is to determine whether there is a difference in the quality of nursing care given to popular and unpopular patients and, if there is, to ascertain whether the difference is measurable as a criterion of the overall quality of nursing care given by a team of nurses to a group of patients.

Two Hypotheses

Arising out of the problem are two *Hypotheses:*
1. That there are some patients whom nurses enjoy caring for and who are more popular than others with nursing staff.
2. That there are observable and measurable differences in the nursing care given to popular and unpopular patients.

In trying to formulate the means of testing these hypotheses, it became apparent that many questions arose which could not be answered by reference to existing theory or from the findings of relevant studies.

Questions

1. Is it possible to determine whether there are some patients who are more popular and some who are less popular than others?
2. If this is so—why?
3. If this is so, are there any reasons in common given for this?
4. Is there an "ideal patient role" that makes a patient enjoyable to to look after?
5. Do deviations from this role make the patient unpopular with the nurses?

Aims

1. To devise a means of identifying popular and unpopular patients in general wards.
2. To identify factors that might account for the popularity and unpopularity of patients.
3. To define the nurses' view of the patient's role.

4. To ascertain whether the degree of popularity influences any aspects of nursing care given to the patients.

Method of Study

1. Rating and ranking techniques for identifying popular and unpopular patients.
2. Analysis of factors that might account for patient unpopularity.
3. Content analysis of the attitudes nurses expressed about their patients.
4. Card sort technique for exploring the nurses' view of the patient's role.
5. A comparative study to gain further information about nurse/patient interaction.

CHAPTER 2

Developing a Tool for Assessing the Popularity and Unpopularity of Patients

Introduction

Many workers have taken an interest in assessing the extent to which members of a group are accepted or rejected by other members and have shown that this can be achieved in one of two ways: either (1) by observation of interaction between all members of the group (it being accepted that where there is a choice and freedom for interaction it will occur with preferred rather than with less preferred members), or (2) by subjective evaluations from the members of the group. In the latter case (*a*) a *forced choice* method may be used, where members of a group are asked to name a stated number of other members they would most and least like to share in a specified area or task, or (*b*) a *free choice* method, where each member is asked to indicate who they would or would not choose to share in a specified area or task. Both methods can have advantages in different situations. The free choice method will indicate the total amount of esteem and disapproval that exists in the group, while the forced choice method is more likely to throw into relief the popular and unpopular members of the group.

Observation of interaction was not the method of choice for this study because in most ward situations nurses do not have choice and freedom for interaction with patients. Tasks may be allocated or "cases" assigned to individual nurses, and the arrangement of beds and the fact that some patients are more mobile than others could influence interaction. It was therefore decided to devise and evaluate the merits of (1) a *free choice rating tool* and (2) a *forced choice ranking tool.*

A Rating Scale for Measuring Popularity

As a criterion of popularity for the rating scale, it was decided to use the nurses' subjective evaluation of how much they enjoyed looking after the patients.

Ideally, at least a five-point scale should be used but it proved impossible to devise a neutral middle sentence, so a four-point scale was devised with the following statements:

   (*a*) I enjoy looking after this patient very much.
   (*b*) I enjoy looking after this patient.
   (*c*) I do not enjoy looking after this patient very much.

(*d*) I do not enjoy looking after this patient.

The nurses were asked to use the appropriate letter to indicate which sentence best applied to each patient in their care. A space was left on the form for recording any reasons of inability to rate a patient (see Appendix 4). The letters were translated into numerical scores, with 4 for sentence (*a*) and 1 for sentence (*d*).

A trial study of the rating scale was carried out in a male surgical ward and a female medical ward in a teaching hospital and a female surgical ward and a female medical ward in a R.H.B. hospital.

It took three days in each ward for all the members of the nursing staff to appear on duty and participate in the trial. In all, 79 patients and 47 nurses took part in this trial study.

Two scores were derived:

1. The *rating score*, being the average rating of each patient made by the nurses, and
2. The *allocation score*, being the average rating of all the patients made by each nurse individually (see Table 1).

TABLE 1

Range of Rating Scores. Allocation Scores and Average Allocation Scores

Ward Composition			Rating Scores received by Patients		Allocation Scores received by Patients		
Ward	Patients	Nurses	Lowest	Highest	Lowest	Highest	Average
1	21	14	2·4	4·0 (2 Pts)	3·0	3·8	3·4
2	21	14	2·1	3·9	3·0	3·9	3·5
3	16	9	3·4	4·0 (3 Pts)	3·6	4·0	3·8
4	21	10	2·5	3·9	3·1	3·9	3·5
Total	79	47					

Subjective observation and evaluation by the researcher of the amount and type of nurse/patient interaction did not corroborate the order of the overall amount of enjoyment expressed by the nurses as measured by the average allocation scores.

The range of scores was too small to be meaningful and some nurses expressed difficulty in recording on paper what amounted to adverse comments about their patients. It was therefore decided, in spite of the fact that the rating method did identify the patients whom the nurses most and least enjoyed caring for, to explore the possibilities of a forced choice ranking method.

A Ranking Scale for Measuring Popularity

For the ranking scale the same criterion of how much the nurses enjoyed looking after the patients was used for an assessment of popularity, as in the rating scale method.

The names of all the patients were written on cards and the nurses were asked to sort these into the order in which, at that time, they enjoyed looking after each patient, with the person they most enjoyed at the top of the pile and the one they least enjoyed at the bottom.

When each nurse had arranged the names in order, an arbitrary score of plus 3, 2 and 1 was given to the three top patients and minus 3, 2 and 1 to the three at the bottom. It was expected that any patient who was particularly popular or unpopular would figure in every nurse's top or bottom three cards. As different numbers of nurses and patients were involved in each ward, a scoring system had to be devised that would take into account the score allocated to each patient in relation to the number of nurses who could contribute to the score. This was achieved by working out each patient's score as a percentage of the highest or lowest score that could have been allocated if they had been placed at the top or bottom by all the nurses; this was termed the percentage ranking score. Thus in ward 5a, for example, 7 nurses took part in the rating. The highest possible score that a patient could get there was $7 \times 3 = 21$; and the lowest possible score a patient could get likewise $7 \times -3 = -21$.

The trial study for this method was carried out in four wards, one of which was administratively divided into two and was therefore treated as two separate entities, making in all five units. The wards were:

A male and female surgical ward, (in two parts), and a female medical ward in a teaching hospital;

A female medical ward and a male surgical ward in a R.H.B. hospital.

Table 2 shows the percentage ranking scores allocated to the most and least popular patient in each ward (cols. 4 and 5). For example the most popular patient in ward 5a was given a score of 20 out of a possible 21 points (95%), the least popular patient was given 11 out of a possible 21 negative points (52%).

The percentage ranking scores suggest that the nurses tend to be in greater agreement about which patients they enjoyed looking after most than about which patients they enjoyed looking after least.

Columns 6 and 7 of the table give the number of patients in each ward who were not placed in the top or bottom three by any nurse, and the number of patients in each ward who were placed in the top three by some nurses and in the bottom three by others.

This method identifies the most and least popular patients in the wards, and the scores give some indication of the extent to which the nurses enjoyed caring for individual patients.

TABLE 2

Percentage Ranking Scores Allocated by the Nurses to the Most and Least
Popular Patients in Each Ward

Ward Composition			Percentage Ranking Scores		Number of Patients with Scores having	
Ward	No. of Patients	No. of Nurses	of the Most Popular Patient	of the Least Popular Patient	No + or −	Both + & −
(1)	(2)	(3)	(4)	(5)	(6)	(7)
5a	15	7	95	52	2	2
5b	16	6	89	39	5	4
6	20	9	41	59	3	4
7	20	6	84	55	6	1
8	15	8	50	50	1	3
Total	86	36			17	14

Both the percentage ranking scores, and the number of patients
given discrepant scores (col. 7) are indications of the extent of the
agreement among nurses about whether or not they enjoyed looking
after individual patients.

One of the advantages of the ranking method is that it is possible to
ask the nurses what criteria they use in making their assessments as to
which patients they most and least enjoy caring for and, since this made
a valuable contribution to the study, it was decided to use the ranking
method.

CHAPTER 3

Testing Factors that Might Account for Unpopularity

This part of the study was based on the assumption that there are no factors other than patients' personality to account for some patients being found unpopular with the nursing team.

The information about patients which it was decided to collect and test was determined in part by theoretical considerations, relating mainly to prejudice and stigma, partly by reference to nursing literature (see Ch. 13), partly by discussion with colleagues and partly by reference to a small study carried out previously at a teaching hospital.

Factors that might affect prejudice towards patients were thought to include age, religion, nationality and social class. Stigmas might occur in relation to certain types of illness, disfigurement, blindness, deafness, obesity, aphasia, dysphasia, confusion and incontinence. The patients' previous acquaintance with hospital wards and the length of their present stay were also considered relevant; terms "hospitalized patient" and "hospital bird" may be used in a derogatory way to describe patients who have been in the ward for some time and whom the nurses do not enjoy looking after. A factor not considered during the early stages of the study but included later was whether a patient was diagnosed as, or suspected of, needing psychiatric treatment.

A rough guide to the patients' personality was attempted by assessing their sociability, in response to questions as to whether they lived with a relative, friend or on their own. (See Appendix 1.)

Two data collection schedules were drawn up for collecting information from patients and nurses (see Appendix 4). The information required from the nurses was essentially the same as that from the patients so that "prejudice factors" could be compared, but this became impossible to analyse.

In the first instance the data was collected from 165 patients and 13 nurses in the same eight wards used for the rating and ranking scales (see Ch. 2 also Tables 1 and 2). Straight counts of the distribution of factors in each category were related to the popularity/unpopularity scorings.

Data from the second study of 223 patients in the four wards in which the later comparative study was carried out (see Chapter 8) was eventually amalgamated with the data of the 165 patients from the eight wards of the initial part of the study, giving a total of 388 patients.

Results

1. Use of popularity rating scales

In the trial study of 79 patients there was a popularity score range of 2·14 to 4. This range was divided into class intervals of 0·1. For analysis the patients with the seven lowest scores (least popular) were compared with the patients with the eight highest scores (most popular) (see Table 3).

TABLE 3

Previous Hospitalization of the Most and Least Popular Patient

Popularity	Previous Hospitalization		Total
	None or Less than 2 weeks	Over 2 weeks	
High score group	6	2	8
Low score group	1	6	7

(p, by exact test, < ·05)

Nearly all the "high group" had not been in hospital before; by contrast nearly all of the "low group" had over two weeks previous hospitalization. The only other area where there was observable difference was that five out of seven of the low scoring group lived on their own, whereas none of the high scoring group did so. (See Appendix 1.)

2. Use of popularity ranking scales

For 86 patients there was a popularity score range of −59% to +95% and for analysis three classes of patients were compared; all the patients with minus scores (37); all those with plus scores (31) and all those with no score (18).

Chi-square tests for significance[1] were carried out where there was any observable difference in the distribution of factors, but none of these were significant beyond the 0·1 level.

3. The combined rating, ranking and comparative study wards

Three different methods were used in evaluating the most and least popular patients in the various wards; the patients were assigned to five classes for assessing the distribution of factors. In the first class were those patients in whom the majority of nurses in any ward in-

---

[1] The Chi-square (X^2) test is a statistical tool, based on laws of probability and sampling, which is used to compare the "observed frequency" of categories of facts with their "expected frequency" and measures the degree to which these frequencies differ. The results are expressed as levels of probability. For example, if $P < 0.05$, the difference between the observed and expected frequencies is said to be statistically significant, and likely to be due to chance less than five times in 100.

dicated their enjoyment in giving care (marked $++$ in the tables); in the second class were those to whom some of the nurses indicated they enjoyed giving care (marked $+$); in the third class were those who did not figure one way or the other (marked 0); in the fourth class were those to whom some of the nurses showed they did not enjoy giving care (marked $-$); in the fifth class were those to whom the majority of nurses indicated they did not enjoy giving care (marked $--$).

TABLE 4

Classification of Patients by Popularity

	Class 1	Class 2	Class 3	Class 4	Class 5	Total
Marking	$++$	$+$	0	$-$	$--$	
No. of Patients	23	49	228	56	32	388
% of Patients	6	13	59	14	8	100%

When patients were classified into five groups in this way no significant relations were found between popularity and age, religious affiliation, social class or home living arrangements (see Appendix 1).

The following tables summarize the factors found to have significant influence on the popularity of patients.

TABLE 5

Popularity of U.K. and Foreign Patients

	Class 1	Class 2	Class 3	Class 4	Class 5	Total
Marking	$++$	$+$	0	$-$	$--$	
Country of origin						
U.K.	22	48	208	47	26	351
Foreign	1	1	20	9	6	37
Totals	23	49	228	56	32	388

When U.K. patients are compared with foreign patients a significantly higher proportion of foreign patients figure in the unpopular classes; and far more of the U.K. patients are popular, $(0.05 > p > 0.02)$.

20

TABLE 6

Classification of Patients by Popularity and Country of Origin

Marking	Class 1 ++		Class 2 +		Class 3 0		Class 4 −		Class 5 −−		Total
Country of origin	Pts	%	Pts	%	Pts	%	Pts	%	Pts	%	
England	22	6	48	14	201	58	47	14	26	8	344
Wales	—		—		3	100	—		—		3
Scotland	—		—		3	100	—		—		3
N/Ireland	—		—		1		—		—		1
Eire	—		—		8	66	2	17	2	17	12
W/Indies	—		—		2	40	2	40	1	20	5
Africa	—		—		—		—		1	100	1
Asia	1	14	—		2	29	3	43	1	14	7
Other	—		1	8	8	67	2	17	1	8	12
Totals	23		49		228		56		32		388

TABLE 7

Classification of Patients by Popularity and Length of Present Stay in Hospital

Length of present Stay in Hospital	Class 1 + +		Class 2 +		Class 3 0		Class 4 —		Class 5 — —		Total
	Pts	%	Pts	%	Pts	%	Pts	%	Pts	%	
< 1 week	5	4	8	6	97	70	22	15	7	5	139
< 1 month	6	14	28	18	88	58	22	14	9	6	153
< 3 months	10	16	9	14	32	50	6	9	7	11	64
< 1 year	2	7	4	14	10	33	6	20	8	27	30
1 year +	—		—		1	50	—		1	50	2
Totals	23	6	49	13	228	59	56	14	32	8	388

When patients in hospital for less than three months are compared with patients in hospital for more than three months, a significantly higher proportion of the longer stay category are classed as unpopular, ($0.01 > p > 0.001$).

TABLE 8

Classification of Patients by Popularity and Length of Previous Stay in Hospital

Length of Previous Stay in Hospital	Class 1 ++		Class 2 +		Class 3 0		Class 4 −		Class 5 − −		Total
	Pts	%	Pts	%	Pts	%	Pts	%	Pts	%	
< 1 week	2	22	2	22	4	44	1	11	—		9
< 1 month	6	8	7	9	48	63	10	13	5	7	76
< 3 months	1	1·5	12	18	37	55	7	10·5	10	15	67
< 1 year	1	3	3	10	17	54	7	23	3	10	31
1 year +	—		—		1	25	1	25	2	50	4
None	11	8	17	12	91	63	21	14	5	3	145
Not Ascertained	2	4	8	14	30	53	9	16	7	13	56
Totals	23	6	49	13	228	59	56	14	32	8	388

When patients with more than three months previous experience of hospital are compared with those with less than three months experience or none, a significantly higher proportion in the unpopular class of patients have had the longer experience of hospital (0·1 > p > 0·05).

TABLE 9

Classification of Patients by Popularity and Defect

(Defects included disfigurement, obesity, deafness, aphasia and psychiatric conditions. Some patients had multiple defects)

	Class 1		Class 2		Class 3		Class 4		Class 5		Total
	Pts	% ++	Pts	% +	Pts	% 0	Pts	% −	Pts	% − −	
Not defective	18	6	39	13	192	64	37	12	16	5	302
Defective	5	5	10	12	36	42	19	22	16	19	86
Totals	23		49		228		56		32		388

Patients with defects were significantly less popular than those without defects, $(p < 0.01)$.

Diagnosis

The range of conditions being too great and the fact that there were many conditions not represented made it impossible to determine whether diagnosis had any influence on the patients' popularity or unpopularity. The only point of interest to emerge was that of 29 patients with a psychiatric diagnosis in the medical and surgical wards none figured in the class of popular patients, 14 were placed in the neutral class and 15 in the unpopular class.

Summary

In testing certain factors which might have bearing on the popularity or unpopularity of patients with the nurses, there was evidence to suggest that foreign patients, those in hospital for more than three months and those with more than three months' previous experience of hospital, and those with some kind of defect, figured significantly in the unpopular group. It also appeared that patients with a psychiatric diagnosis (including those who were admitted following a suicidal attempt) were more likely to be found unpopular than popular, although it was not possible to submit this particular factor to significance tests, as questions on it had not been included in the particulars collected about the patients.

CHAPTER 4

Nurses' Attitudes Towards Patients

In the four wards where the ranking method of identifying popular and unpopular patients was carried out (see p. 16), the nurses were asked to write down their reasons for placing their particular choices at the top and the bottom of their ranking scale.

On one side of a sheet of paper was the statement:
"You have indicated that you most enjoy looking after .... in this ward. Please would you give your reasons for making this choice. It is important that your reasons should be as truthful as possible and anything you write will be completely confidential."

When the nurse had completed this side the paper was turned over to show the statement:
"You have also indicated that the patient you least enjoy looking after is .... Please would you give your reasons for making this choice.

A total of 36 nurses in the four wards completed the forms (there were no refusals). All of them gave two or more reasons for choosing the patient they most enjoyed caring for and altogether there were 120 comments.

Twenty-eight nurses gave two or more reasons for choosing the patient they least enjoyed looking after. Of the eight who made only one comment five gave such reasons as that they were too well to need nursing or too recently admitted to be known; one nurse said she only enjoyed looking after the interesting cases and of the other patients it was just chance which one she placed last. A total of 70 comments were made by the 36 nurses.

For the analysis each comment was treated as a separate entity although in most cases there were several comments about each patient and some patients were chosen by more than one nurse.

Results

A content analysis was made from the collected material and the comments fell roughly into four main categories.
1. Personality factors, e.g. cheerful, pleasant, selfish, bad-tempered.
2. Communication factors, e.g. grateful, amusing, uncooperative, grumbling.
3. Attitude factors, e.g. understanding, optimistic, unwilling to accept treatment, reluctant to go home.

4. Nursing factors, e.g. interesting to nurse, needs nursing, does not need to be in hospital, not well known.

It was appreciated that communication factors and attitude factors are closely related to personality but it was felt that there was some value in making the distinction.

In addition to the written comments further information was collected from the nurses working in the four wards where the comparative study was carried out (see Chapter 7). During that part of the study 36 nurses were interviewed and were asked to rank the patients in the order in which they enjoyed looking after them and were then asked to give the reasons for their choice verbally. These comments (163) were analysed in the same way as the written comments.

Table 10 summarizes the classified distribution of reasons given by two groups of different nurses for enjoying or not enjoying looking after patients. A fuller account of the comments appears in Appendix 2.

TABLE 10

Distribution of Reasons Given by Two Groups of Different Nurses for Enjoying or Not Enjoying Looking after Patients

	Reasons for Enjoying		Reasons for Not Enjoying	
	Written %	Verbal %	Written %	Verbal %
Personality factors	33	30	36	34
Communication factors	32	45	38	31
Attitude factors	16	13	10	7
Nursing factors[1]	19	12	16	28
Total %	100	100	100	100

[1] These figures include 19 unclassified items such as "vulgar", "boring", "fussy", which should be represented under personality factors.

Summary

From a total of 353 favourable and unfavourable comments only 34 (9·6%) were completely unrelated to personality factors and in all but four instances there were additional references to personality included in the statement. It would seem therefore that this analysis of the nurses' comments tends to support the assumption that there are no factors other than personality to account for some patients being found unpopular by the nursing team.

CHAPTER 5

Exploring the Nurses' View of the Patients' Role

Introduction

The theoretical considerations on which this study is based (see Ch. 11) indicate that in any group situation members are assigned positions conferring certain rights and obligations on them and these are termed roles. The rights and obligations of any particular role are defined by members of the immediate group, by other groups that impinge on the situation and by cultural factors. Pressures are brought to bear on individuals who do not comply with their defined role, firstly to encourage them to conform and then, if this is of no avail, to attempt to ostracize them. The role definers in any given situation have power to exercise both rewarding and punishing sanctions, and conversely, the people with power in any situation have the most authority to define roles.

In a ward situation nurses have power in relationship to the patients and so, in theory, will play a large part in defining the patients' role in the ward. It is to be expected that patients who do not conform to their defined role will be less liked than those who do. The same is true of the patients in that, being the "raison d'etre" of the ward, they have a certain amount of intrinsic power and will contribute to a definition of the nurses' role, preferring those who conform to those who do not.

There are many facets in any particular role and the weight attached to these will vary with regard to the necessity to conform to them. For example, as Talcott Parsons (1964) points out, in acute wards it is accepted that patients should want to get well and should therefore cooperate to this end. If any patient is seen to have a good chance of recovery but does not wish to get well, the discomfort this brings to those caring for him is easy to observe. On the other hand, it may be a rule that patients are not allowed in the kitchen but in some situations willing helpers may even be encouraged to go in.

In any given ward situation there will be some aspects of the patient's role that are similar to those in other situations and some that will be peculiar to that ward.

In developing a way of defining the nurse's view of the patient's role the common denominator factors should become apparent and the areas in which specific factors are defined should be revealed.

It was felt that it would be unwise to test this method with the nurses who were being asked to state their feelings about the patients they enjoyed and did not enjoy caring for, since their overall view of the patients' behaviour was likely to be coloured by the particular individuals upon whom their attention was focused. It was therefore decided to seek the cooperation of nursing staff in wards adjacent to the one where the popularity study was being carried out, and where this was not feasible some of the student nurses in the training school were asked to participate. Some nurses who were attending courses at the Royal College of Nursing also participated and in all 34 nurses contributed to this part of the study.

In order not to miss the opportunity, a questionnaire, with 12 statements chosen at random from many possibilities was given to the nurses participating in the ranking scale popularity study (see Appendix 3(b)). This was done with the idea of determining whether their responses reflected their verbalized choices of most and least liked patients. This analysis was not, in fact, carried out because the statements did not adequately reflect the nurses' comments. The results of the responses by 38 nurses to the 12 statements are given in Appendix 3(b).

Development of the Role Definition Tool

In order to get the nurses' opinions it was decided to type a variety of statements about patients' behaviour on cards and ask the nurses to sort them into five categories of: Strongly agree; agree; do not know; disagree; strongly disagree.

The statements were based on references to the literature, discussion with colleagues, personal observation and information collected earlier in the study.

Among a total of 44 statements each item was paired, as far as possible, with one that expressed the same sentiment in an opposite or different way. For example:

"I do not like it when patients tell tales about each other", and "I want patients to tell me if other patients are breaking the rules."

In this way it was hoped to provide an internal check on individual consistency.

The cards were well shuffled before each nurse sorted them. Some statements were worded positively and others negatively. It was evident while listening to comments made by the nurses when sorting the cards that they sometimes had difficulty in putting a negative statement with which they agreed on an "agree" pile. For example, they might say, "I do not like it when patients tell tales about each other—no, I do not," and then placed it on the "disagree" pile, whereas in fact, they agreed with the statement while disagreeing with the sentiment. For this reason some of the negatively worded sentences were changed to positively worded ones.

29

After a nurse had sorted the statements, the responses were charted and the evolving pattern of agreement, disagreement and conflicting opinion was observed. Where there were a lot of "do not know" responses and also some division of opinion, the sentences were slightly reworded and tried on the next group of nurses. Any comments the nurses made to themselves or to the observer were given consideration and this led to some of the sentences being reworded or discarded and replaced by others.

Results

The card sorting tool that attempted to define the nurse's view of the patient's role was not used with a large enough sample of nurses to achieve this aim. The full list of statements and responses to them are given in Appendix 3(*a*).

Of the 44 statements made only seven showed the participants to be in complete agreement or disagreement. Five of these showed complete agreement:

1. It makes nursing much easier when patients are cheerful.
2. I always welcome patients' offers to help me if they are well enough to do so.
3. I think patients should help themselves as much as they can.
4. I like patients who make every effort to get better quickly.
5. I think patients like helping with jobs on the ward.

The two showing complete disagreement were:

6. I want patients to tell me if other patients are breaking the rules.
7. I think patients should be allowed their own way while they are in hospital.

The two statements in the 12 item questionnaire that elicited most concurrence were:

1. The more experience that patients have had of hospital, the easier they are to look after—30 out of 38 nurses disagreed.
2. A tidy patient is a godsend—29 out of 38 nurses agreed.

A list of the statements and responses is given in Appendix 3(*b*).

Summary of Part I

This part of the study has shown that it is possible to identify patients who are popular and unpopular with the nurses. Among factors likely to account for unpopularity were foreign nationality and a stay in hospital of over three months, also patients with a psychiatric diagnosis.

The role definition tool that it was hoped to formulate was not refined enough to discriminate between one nurse's view and another's because the essential role factors were not identified.

At this stage it was felt necessary to obtain more information about interpersonal behaviour in the ward situation at source and so a different technique was adopted and a comparative study undertaken which is outlined in Part II.

PART II

CHAPTER 6

Comparative Analysis Defined

The comparative method of analysis is used in the field of social anthropology where a society may be studied in depth and the observed behaviours compared with the stated norms of another society or where several societies are studied to establish the behaviours and patterns of interaction occurring in each society and those that are unique to any one of them.

From these observations theoretical constructs may be hypothesized which will be faithful to the everyday realities of the situation and can be tested under experimental conditions.

Nadel (1951) *The Foundation of Social Anthropology* describes the aim of the comparative method as being to demonstrate the extent to which uniformities or differences in any one feature are accompanied by uniformities or differences in others. He states that this method presupposes three things: first, some preliminary hypothesis or suspicion as to the kind of correlation likely to prove relevant; secondly, the method implies the general postulate that social situations are not made up of random items but of facts which hang together in some meaningful nexus or intrinsic "fitness"; thirdly, judgements have to be made on the identity and difference of social facts. These judgements must be such that there can be general agreement about them.

Merton (1957) with what he describes as functional analysis, relates the comparative process to the sociological field. For him a function, in relation to sociology, is a vital or organic process in which individual beings, "the essential units", are connected by networks of social relations into an integrated whole. It is also the part played by any recurrent activity in the social life as a whole with its contribution to the maintenance of structural continuity. The theoretical framework of a functional analysis must, therefore, expressly require that there be specification of the "units" for which a given social or cultural item is functional, and must also allow for a given item having diverse consequences, functional and dysfunctional, for individuals, for subgroups and for the more inclusive social structure and culture.

Glaser and Strauss (1968) also relate the comparative method to the sociological field and they describe a process of generating theory by using what they term the constant comparative method. This comprises

31

formulating a tentative theory and then listing all the relevant conceptual elements which they term "categories". Observations are then recorded in various situations and incidents applicable to each category are recorded. A "property" is defined as being a conceptual aspect of a category and, as observations proceed, categories and their properties are integrated to make some theoretical sense of each comparison. New categories are included and new theory evolves to accord with the findings during the process of observation.

CHAPTER 7

Aims and Method of Comparison for this Study

The previous stages of the study showed that there was not enough information available about such topics as the nurses' view of the patients' role and patterns of nurse/patient interaction to be able to continue usefully without further information. Also for the underlying purpose of the Project, which was to devise means of measuring the quality of nursing care, observations of nurse/patient interaction were needed in order to determine the possibility of measuring any differences in nursing care related to ensuring that patients' emotional needs were being met.

The aims of the comparative study were therefore:

1. To gain information about the nurses' view of the patients' role.
2. To explore further what factors accounted for the popularity and unpopularity of patients with the nurses.
3. To observe what factors influenced the amount and type of nurse/patient interaction.
4. To ascertain the extent to which patients' emotional needs were being met.

Methods

1. *Non-participant selective observation*

All the observations were recorded by the researcher. Patients and nurses were referred to by code numbers and observations of incidents, conversations and comments relevant to the aims of the study were recorded briefly at the time or shortly after they were made and were expanded and categorized after leaving the ward for the day.

Observations were made of the day staff only, with an approximately eight-hour period spent in the ward each day, the hours being varied in time to cover the different shifts. The staff of the ward were told that the researcher was studying interpersonal relationships in the ward situation.

In all the wards it was impossible to observe the whole area from any one vantage point and so it was decided in advance which particular aspect was to be the focus for the day. The researcher then either stayed in one position and observed anything relevant that occurred in the visible area or moved around to be where the relevant things were happening. It is fair to assume that the people being observed were for the most part aware of the researcher's presence.

2. *Data collection from nurses and patients*

The data collection schedules that were developed for the earlier part of the study were completed for all the patients and nurses who spent time in the ward during the period of observation.

Some of the nursing factors (see Appendix 4, item 18, of the patients' schedule) were difficult to record, as over a period of three or four weeks the situation could change. Thus, if at any point during the period of observation any of the nursing factor items applied, they were recorded, but if a nurse made any comment about her own attitude in relation to the appearance or disappearance of any nursing item, this was also recorded.

The patients' schedules were completed from the nursing records, case notes and by conversation with the patients. The nurses' schedules were completed during their interview with the observer.

3. *Assessment of popular and unpopular patients*

The ranking method developed during the earlier stages of the study was used. Each nurse was asked to rank the patients once only during the period of observation and all the patients who had been in the ward or were still there were included among the cards for sorting. If there was any patient the nurse had not met or could not remember, the card was put aside. The scoring was complicated by the fact that some nurses did their ranking early in the observation period and some later, so that each nurse was ranking a slightly different population of patients. In spite of these drawbacks patterns of likes and dislikes emerged, while changes in the patterns became apparent to the observer through listening to reporting sessions and to the nurses' comments.

During the interview, the nurses were asked to give their reasons for the highest and lowest rankings; these responses are set out in Chapter 3 and Appendix 2.

4. *Semi-structured interviews with the nurses*

Individual interviews were conducted in privacy somewhere in the ward and lasted from over half to three-quarters of an hour.

At some point during the observation periods 44 nursing staff were interviewed in the four wards. The time available for interview was sometimes too short for the nurse to be able to rank the patients and eight nurses were asked instead to name the patients they most and least enjoyed caring for. Fifteen nurses were not interviewed either because they left the ward too early, came to work in the ward too late, or because they were on sick leave.

The topics covered in the interview were introduced in a fairly random order, except that the question about ideal and least ideal patients did not immediately follow the discussion about most and least liked patients currently in the ward.

The interview topics were as follows:

1. The process of ranking the patients according to how much the nurses enjoyed looking after them.
2. Reasons for ranking the highest and lowest and comments about any other patients in the ward.
3. Reasons for taking up nursing.
4. How preconceptions about nursing compare with reality.
5. Attitudes to nursing in general.
6. Attitudes to the present ward in comparison with others they have worked in.
7. What they had heard about the ward before coming to work there.
8. The pleasures and rewards they find in nursing.
9. Their dislikes in nursing.
10. An inquiry as to what they understood by the emotional needs of patients.
11. Their concept of an ideal patient.
12. Their concept of the least ideal patient.
13. Questions or further comments.

CHAPTER 8

The Choice of Wards

A decision had to be reached about how many situations it would be profitable to use for meaningful comparisons to be made. Time and cost limited the total number of wards that could be included but enough diversity was needed so that events which occurred in common could stand out, and enough similarity so that unique events could be identified.

It was originally intended to study two medical and two surgical wards, one of each in a teaching and a R.H.B. hospital. In the event the time allowed at the teaching hospital proved insufficient to study two wards, and the surgical ward was therefore omitted. At the R.H.B. hospital the method of progressive patient care through different wards was practised with the surgical patients and because it was felt that the resulting lack of continuity of care would not be suitable for this stage of the study, a geriatric ward was substituted to provide a contrast. Finally, to make up the fourth ward, a medical ward at another teaching hospital was included.

The matron or her deputy chose the wards in which the study would be carried out and on each occasion they were chosen because they were considered to be good of their kind. "Good" in each case of the medical wards meant they were efficiently and well run and one was also judged "good" because nurses requested to work there when they qualified. The geriatric ward was considered good because the patients were physically well cared for.

Requests at two of the hospitals to be allocated a high and low morale ward were on both occasions firmly rejected.

For ease of description the four wards were given the following pseudonyms:

1. ASH WARD. A medical ward in a teaching hospital for male and female patients.
2. ELM WARD. A medical ward in a R.H.B. hospital for men.
3. FIR WARD. A female geriatric ward in a R.H.B. hospital.
4. OAK WARD. A male medical ward in a teaching hospital.

CHAPTER 9

Portraits of the Wards

ASH WARD

Geography

This was a mixed medical ward that had recently been reconstructed and redecorated. Four separate bed areas contained beds for 18 women, one of them being in a cubicle; seven men, one of them in a cubicle; and four for male staff with medical or surgical conditions.

The nurses' station was partitioned off from the women's area on one side of the ward and the treatment room was off the other side. The kitchen was between the two on the treatment room side and, having two doors, provided a way through, but because of the inconvenience to the domestic staff this was not allowed and a chain was put across one door. The other door into the ward on that side was at the far end of the larger bed area and often necessitated quite a detour. The sister's office, the patients' sitting room, the nurses' changing room, also various medical and secretarial staff offices and some storage cupboards were on an upstairs level, reached by two staircases leading from the women's wards on either side of the corridor.

Because of the arrangement of the ward it was often difficult to find a particular person as the staff were constantly on the move. On the other hand it was easy to get "lost" if there were no tasks to be done. A complicating factor was the triple arrangement of telephones, with internal and external phones in the nurses' station, beside the treatment room and in the sister's office upstairs. The outside line was a joint one and could be answered at any point but it was impossible to see if anyone was moving to answer it elsewhere.

Another problem caused by the planning of the ward was that patients in the sitting room felt very isolated and rarely used it unless they could join others and go up as a group.

Nursing Staff

During the period of observation 16 nurses of varying grades worked in the ward on day duty. The night nurses were allocated to the ward separately.

The ward sister had worked there for about six years and the senior part-time staff nurse for nearly a year. On the day the observation period started, three of the nurses obtained their State Final results; the two that had passed appeared in their staff nurses' uniform for the first time and were staying in the ward until they had decided what to do next.

There were seven student nurses and four pupil nurses. One of the student nurses was seconded from a psychiatric hospital for three months' experience. A German girl was working in the ward as a nursing auxiliary on a year's exchange scheme.

The majority of the nursing staff were English, with one from Trinidad and one from Jamaica.

Ward Organization

The nursing staff mainly worked straight shifts but occasionally someone had to work a split shift.

The nurses on duty were divided into two teams, each looking after half the ward. The half in which any nurse worked was allocated arbitrarily and could vary from day to day. The nurses themselves arranged who did which tasks; there was a list of routine work and a day book which indicated any special treatments or tests for individual patients. The sister and staff nurses used a "change book" to record changes in treatment, requests for X-ray and other services and items to be remembered. This book was available to the nurses for reference.

Leadership, Relationships and Communications

In discussion, the ward sister expressed concern about the difficulty of ensuring efficiency by constantly checking up and nagging, while still maintaining a free atmosphere in which the patients could feel happy and the nurses enjoyed working.

In practice, the sister appeared to be easy-going and friendly towards the senior nurses but checked and chased the juniors. She delegated most of the routine administrative tasks and responsibility for supervising the juniors to the staff nurses, while still remaining in command of the situation. Much of her time was spent in attending ward rounds, since beds were assigned to six consultants, but this also provided opportunity to observe the nurses and to ensure that routine observations had been made and recorded.

When the sister was off duty or on sick leave, there was no change in the atmosphere of the ward. The staff nurses respected her authority and yet had a friendly relationship with her and felt she would listen to any suggestions they might make. The student nurses felt she was fair, but some had heard before coming to the ward that she could be very cross if she found anyone slacking. One nurse said, "you untidy the sluice so you can tidy it again" and another remarked, "you can make things like the medicine round last a long time". All the nurses except one pupil nurse and the German auxiliary felt it would be regarded as "slacking" just to chat to patients, but another recalled with pleasure that on one occasion the sister had told her to go and talk to a particular patient.

The nurses seemed friendly towards each other and were mostly on Christian name terms. The pupil nurses, most of whom were doing combined trainings with other hospitals, commented particularly on the friendliness in the ward; they also expressed appreciation for being allowed to do what they called "the proper jobs" such as dressings and helping with medicine rounds.

The housemen, whom the sister and senior nurses addressed and referred to by their Christian names, joined in the friendly interaction on the ward.

Nurses coming on day duty read the report from the Kardex and at 9 a.m. the sister or a staff nurse gave them a report in the upstairs office, which provided opportunity for teaching. Questions and observations from the students were encouraged and although, if asked, they would say what they had noticed, they did not really feel that their observations were very welcome. They supposed that the sister and staff nurses noticed more than anyone else what was going on and felt that their own observations might be interpreted as criticism. As one nurse said, "You are taught to report things you notice, but you don't often do it, except with things like dressings that you know Sister has not seen".

ELM WARD

Geography

This was a permanent hutted ward redecorated and modified three years previously and used for male medical patients. The modifications and improvements included a four bed bay for a coronary unit, a day room shared with the next ward, and better bathroom and toilet facilities.

The 21 beds in the ward were under the care of one consultant physician, but a consultant with beds in the adjacent ward sometimes had patients in the coronary unit until they were well enough to be moved.

The first two cubicles on either side of the entrance corridor were partitioned with wood and opaque glass with sliding doors. The next cubicle on either side was a curtained space between the cubicle and coronary unit partition. A two-bedded bay on each side made up the coronary unit having curtained cubicles within wood and clear glass partitions. The remaining 11 beds were arranged Nightingale fashion in the open ward.

The day room, off the corridor leading to the adjacent ward, was a large room with french windows, much glass and no door separating it from the corridor. Consequently it was rather draughty in winter and, although used as a television viewing room, the patients mostly preferred to sit in the ward area.

Nursing Staff

During the period of observation 15 nurses and a ward clerk worked in the ward on day duty. No more than 10 nurses were allocated to the ward at any one time, including the ward sister. The night nurses were allocated separately.

The sister had been promoted two months previously having already worked in the ward as a staff nurse for about eight months. Her deputy was a nurse undergoing a further training period having failed her State Registration finals three times elsewhere. Of the rest, none of whom were qualified, nine were students, one was a pupil, one was a cadet and two were nursing auxiliaries. Six of the nurses were English, five were from Eire and one from Northern Ireland, one came from Canada, one from Hong Kong and one from Malaysia.

Ward Organization

All the nurses worked straight shifts.

Organization of the ward work was done entirely by word of mouth. There was no list of routine care, no list of special investigations or treatments (apart from a medicine list) and no individual work list. Some items were mentioned in the Kardex but not all, and dates and instructions for some tests were pinned on the board above the sister's desk. The students themselves arranged who should do which tasks and on the whole they did things together as far as possible.

Leadership, Relationships and Communications

The ward sister had nursed abroad for some time and she expressed concern that the nurses seemed to show so little interest in finding out things about the patients and never seemed to ask questions. She realized that, without any staff nurses, she had to spend quite a lot of time on administrative tasks and could not therefore see as much of the patients or the nurses as she would like. In her relationships with the nurses and doctors she was very formal, although she had worked as a staff nurse with some of the senior student nurses and knew their Christian names, she never used these when speaking to them.

When the sister was off duty the student nurses who were left in charge did not seem very sure of themselves and this lack of confidence was somewhat reflected in the rest of the team. The sister could always be reached by telephone if they wanted help, but it was usually the houseman who was contacted first and often before all the relevant information he would need had been collected.

All the nurses got on well together with the exception of one who was rather aloof and whom the others reported to the sister for not pulling her weight. The other students, especially the ones from abroad, commented on how much more friendly the nurses were in the ward than in the nurses' home. One of the patients commented on how well the nurses of all nationalities pulled together as a team. The juniors said they enjoyed working in this particular ward because they could ask the senior nurses anything they wanted. They did not however include the sister in this category and did not pass on patients' queries to her even when it was likely that she was the only person with the necessary information.

The nurses read the Kardex when they came on duty, and at 11 a.m. when the second shift came on, the ward sister or nurse in charge usually gave a report to all the nurses in the treatment room, leaving observation of the ward to the ward maid.

Because of the off-duty pattern, the sister sometimes did not see her deputy before taking her day off; this necessitated lengthy written communication in order to give information and try to forestall any eventualities that might arise.

Most of the nursing observations were recorded directly on the patients' charts, but there was a book for the twice daily temperatures. The nurses only knew who was having four-hourly observations by the type of chart at the end of the bed. The nurses were required to collect four-hourly print-out records from the patients whose heart function was being monitored, but this was frequently omitted or the records were found to be without the patient's name or the time of recording, or both; constant reminders from the ward sister did not seem to result in improvement.

FIR WARD

Geography

This was a women's geriatric ward in the same hospital as Elm Ward, one of two such wards in the hospital. It was situated on the first floor and was reached by two narrow stair-cases. There was no lift except for a small hoist in the kitchen.

The bed areas were in two wings with three beds in an open area between them; bathrooms with toilets adjacent were at the far ends of the two wings. The commode stands were kept in the bathroom areas and bedpans for these stands were kept in the sluices, both of which were situated in the central area between the two wings. There was one hoist for the whole ward, kept in one or other bathroom.

The 30 beds in the ward were under the care of one consultant, whose aim was to use them in the early stages of rehabilitation for the elderly who had become incontinent, or who had pressure sores or some other physical ailment. A few patients were being cared for on a long-term basis and some were severely demented. The sister tried to put the more demented and incontinent patients together in one wing, while the three most mobile patients slept in the three-bedded area, and spent the day sitting at the end of one of the wards, where there was a limited space and a television set.

Nursing Staff

The number of nurses allocated to this ward varied considerably from week to week as geriatric nursing experience is compulsory for the pupil nurses training both at this hospital and at another in the same group. At the time of the study 14 nurses were allocated to the ward for day duty, including five married women who lived locally and worked part-time, one being an S.E.N. and the others nursing auxiliaries. These five were English and of the student and pupil nurses three were English, one Irish, one Canadian, three Malaysian and one Nigerian.

The sister had been appointed some eight years previously and had also worked in the ward for some years as a staff nurse. One of the nursing auxiliaries had worked in the ward for eight years and in the sister's absence was the most knowledgeable about ward affairs. In the absence of a staff nurse, a student nurse would officially be in charge when the sister was off duty.

Ward Organization

There was no list of ward routine or work list for the nurses and, in practice, the team on duty would start the washings, back rounds, bedpan and commode rounds at the far end of one wing and then work through to the far end of the other. They worked in pairs and as far as possible the auxiliaries, pupils and students paired with one of their own kind. There appeared to be no choice as to who cared for which patients and when they finished one patient the nurses moved to the next one who had not been attended to. This system of working meant that all nursing staff were in one wing at a time, leaving the other wing unsupervised.

As many patients as possible were out of bed in the day time. They could not be dressed as there was no storage space for clothes, but everyone had a bedside locker for her personal possessions.

Leadership, Relationships and Communications

The sister had worked in the hospital and in the ward for many years; like the part-time nurses, she lived locally and knew the area well. Since the ward served the local area, she knew some of the patients before they were admitted and the background of many of the others. Much of this information she did not share with the students or pupil nurses. They were allowed to read the patients' notes and a Kardex nursing record which was kept for some of the patients, but there were no reporting sessions. The student nurses expressed great appreciation if the sister did at any time tell them anything of a patient's background because, as one of them said, "You see them more as a person if you know what they were once". This applied particularly to the demented patients. The pupil nurses, few of whom spoke English, knew practically nothing about the patients, not even their names. All the student and pupil nurses found the work wearying and, while the student nurses found some rewards in the demands it made on them, all the pupils disliked working in the ward and found it very unrewarding.

OAK WARD

Geography

This was a men's medical ward with a total of 31 beds; two were in single rooms, three in a side ward and the rest in the main ward, which was divided into two parts by a structural partition. The two parts were on different levels being joined on one side of the partition by a fairly steep ramp and on the other side by four steps.

The kitchen and a bathroom were at the far end of the lower level, while two toilets used by all the patients, the sluice, the treatment room and another bathroom were situated adjacent to the top level. There was a gas fire in each ward area, around which easy chairs were placed.

Nursing Staff

The number of nurses allocated to the ward fluctuated greatly over the four week observation period. Altogether 20 nurses were in the ward for some of the study period, although in the fourth week there were fewer student nurses than the sister could ever remember. There were four staff nurses, each of whom took it in turns to spend three months on night duty in the ward. The rest of the night staff were allocated separately. Apart from the sister and staff nurses, all the other nursing staff were students at various stages of training; a ward clerk worked on weekdays from nine to five o'clock.

The sister had been in the ward for about three years and all the nurses were English.

Ward Organization

The staff nurses and students worked straight shifts; the sister quite often worked a split shift, mainly because she preferred it. The staff were organized in two teams to care for the patients in the lower and upper level areas. The teams remained fairly fixed although the students sometimes changed from one to another during their stay on the ward. As the beds for the six consultants who had patients in the ward were segregated into the different areas, it meant that the nursing experience was different for each team. There was a list of general routine work and each nurse had tasks allocated for the day.

Leadership, Relationships and Communications

The sister was a strict disciplinarian who was quick to reprimand the nurses if anything was forgotten, or if they were untidy or unpunctual. Several of the senior student nurses commented on the fact that she did not delegate much responsibility to the staff nurses, although only one of the staff nurses mentioned this. Lack of authority on the part of the staff nurses was apparent and this was mentioned by several patients during a few days when the sister was on sick leave. Several of the nurses and many of the patients commented on the sister's nursing ability and powers of observation.

The student nurses worked amicably together, but seemed particularly friendly only with others of the same seniority. At one point five nurses in the same set were allocated to the ward and several made favourable comments about this, such as "This ward's fine at the moment, because several of my friends are here. There are four others in my set, so there's always one of them on duty".

Although the ward had the reputation of being very busy and morbid, the majority of the nurses were enjoying it more than they thought they would, because it was well organized, the reporting sessions were good and they knew what was expected of them.

The nurses read the Kardex reports on starting duty in the morning at 9 a.m. and the sister reported to the staff nurses. Reports were given to the two teams after lunch, and to any nurses coming on duty at 4.30 p.m., either by the sister or a staff nurse. At these sessions, which included teaching, questioning and contributions from the nurses were encouraged.

CHAPTER 10

Four Wards Compared

Observations of the patients' role in the wards

In order to gain more information about the nurses' view of the patients' role in hospital wards, it was accepted by the researcher that people who conform to group norms will be more liked than those who do not, therefore the patients that the nurses most and least enjoyed caring for were identified and their behaviour observed. An attempt was made both through observation and questioning to ascertain what sanctions the nurses employed to reward conforming behaviour and to deter non-conforming behaviour; but subjective evaluation had, of necessity, to play a large part in this.

When nurses changed their opinion of how much they enjoyed looking after patients, an attempt was made to find out what influenced this change.

Finally the nurses' descriptions of their opinion of ideal and least ideal patients were examined and compared with the observations made in the ward by the author.

Behaviour of popular patients

In each of the wards there were one or more patients who were particularly able to communicate with nurses in passing, usually with some sort of cheering or light-hearted remark, and they all ranked high in the nurses' enjoyment of caring for them. In **Ash Ward** the patient most able to do this was a young woman who had been in and out of hospital a lot and on this occasion had been in for six weeks. She was confined to bed, but was situated nearest to the nurses' station. She knew the nurses by name and took an interest in their doings. She also had a small daughter who was brought to visit her every day and this helped to provide a focus of interest and an excuse for stopping at her bedside.

In **Elm Ward** the patient the nurses most enjoyed looking after was a man who had been very ill, but who was then up and about. His work had brought him into contact with hospitals and he liked to think he was familiar with the ways of ward life but was fairly discreet in communicating this to the nurses. On occasion he would tell the junior nurses what to do and this detracted from his popularity with them. He was the centre of the up-patient group and was very helpful to the patients and the nurses would go to him to borrow a watch with a second

45

hand if they were without one. Much of the interaction he initiated was in a bantering or jocular tone and this meant that his occasional expressions of anxiety were not taken seriously, but he circumvented this by arranging for his wife to see the consultant about his worries. Incidentally, this led to several patients doing the same thing.

The most popular patient in **Fir Ward** was a woman who was mobile and independent. She was only occasionally spontaneously talkative, but she always looked up in a friendly way as the nurses went by and laughed if they joked with her or nearby patients and she was willing to do small jobs if asked. Another patient who was very popular in this ward was an old lady who was very demented, very deaf and almost blind, but in her demented state she was perpetually having tea parties and the nurses were identified as friends from the past and invited to join her. They would play up to her delusions, pretending to be the duchess of this and that and they found her very amusing.

As **Oak Ward** was divided into two parts for nursing administration the nurses were ranking two different groups of patients, but there was one patient who had been placed in both areas and was known to all the nurses and they all enjoyed looking after him. He had been resuscitated following three episodes of cardiac arrest and, although he was somewhat apprehensive, this was appreciated by the nurses and was counterbalanced by his good sense of humour and great determination to get well again. In a quiet and undemanding way he always had a word for the nurses as they passed his bed.

Other patients whom the nurses indicated they enjoyed looking after shared these attributes of being able to facilitate communications and approach life in the ward with humour. The other things that these patients, apart from those in the geriatric ward, had in common was that they were all recovering from or showing remission during a fairly severe degree of illness and were able to express gratitude for this.

Summary

Patients the nurses enjoyed caring for:
Were able to communicate readily with the nurses.
Knew the nurses' names.
Were able to joke and laugh with the nurses.
Cooperated in being helped to get well and expressed determination to do so.

Behaviour of "least" popular patients

The patients whom the nurses indicated they did not enjoy looking after fell into two main groups. There were those who indicated that they were not happy to be in the ward, or with what was being done for them, by grumbling and complaining or otherwise demanding attention. In the second group were those whom the nurses felt did not need to be in hospital, or should not be in that particular ward, and whose personalities did not outweigh this judgement.

Two of the patients in **Ash Ward** fitted into the "grumbling" category: both were rather lonely widows and one of them was heard to say how embarrassing it was never having any visitors. Both were overtly self-pitying and found more than their present predicament and the ward to grumble about. One of them did not appear to be particularly miserable, although she had a reputation with most of the nurses for being a grumbler and moaner. On one occasion however, she indulged in some fairly aggressive teasing, as when she was being given her tablets she said to her neighbour "I'm going to shoot this nurse!" and the nurse replied "You can't get guns on the National Health", which elicited the response "Well it will have to be poison then—slow poison". Another patient whom the nurses did not enjoy looking after was a woman very crippled with rheumatoid arthritis. She did not grumble, but she became very cross and sarcastic when frustrated either by being kept waiting for assistance or when a nurse was called away in the middle of doing something for her. She commented to the observer that she was always left until last by the nurses and quoted them as saying, when they eventually came to put her to bed "We've come to do old nuisance now".

Two patients whom the nurses did not enjoy looking after also fitted into the second group. One was a man, admitted in a semi-conscious state following an overdose of barbiturate, who was categorized as being "psychy" and elicited quite a lot of positively expressed hostility from the nurses. He was extremely restless and antagonistic while semi-conscious and he was rather frightening. A seconded psychiatric nurse said she could not get near him "because the other nurses make him so aggressive". It was a fellow patient who stayed by him, calmed him and eventually persuaded him to drink. On regaining consciousness he was very apologetic and ingratiatingly docile, but, as one nurse said, "I must admit, I haven't spoken to him since he came round and I don't want to. You don't know whether to pretend you don't expect him to hit you or to keep well clear in case".

Another patient in the second group was a West Indian woman whom the nurses suspected of malingering. She had been admitted for investigation of possible hypertension, found to have nothing that warranted treatment and was discharged home. Within 24 hours she was back again, having fainted in the street. In the ward she lay unhappily in bed, resisting attempts to encourage her to sit up or get up. The "encouragement" given by the nurses was rather half-hearted and she was described as "a misery who is only homesick and won't help herself ".

In **Elm Ward** there was very little overt grumbling but this was the ward where the patients indulged in the most "jocular grumbling" among themselves, mainly about the food, the cold (especially in the sitting room) and being disturbed by the nurses during their rest hour after lunch. Sometimes the nurses were intended to hear the exchanges, but they would take up the humour aspect, ignoring the underlying complaint. So, in this ward, the two patients whom the nurses least enjoyed caring for were in the group of those not needing to be in hospital. Both these patients had diabetes which was being controlled by diet and they both tested their own specimens and charted the results. The older of the two men was described by the nurses as being lazy and helpless because "he just lies around on his bed all day". On several occasions he complained of the cold to his neighbour but he did not communicate this to the nurses. The other patient did not think he should be in hospital and was reluctant either to test his urine specimens (sometimes guessing the results), or to keep to his diet, though the nurses did not seem to be aware of this. The fact that he continually expressed a desire to be away from the place and chivvied the doctors to discharge him seemed to make the nurses very disinterested in his welfare and progress.

The patients the nurses least enjoyed caring for in **Fir Ward** were two women, diagnosed since admission as having endogenous depression, both of whom were volitionally retarded, looked miserable and did not appear to be making any progress. There was also a woman with severe dementia who had contracture deformities and was very noisy and physically aggressive when the nurses attended her.

In **Oak Ward** the man the nurses most positively did not enjoy caring for did not have a stated diagnosis. He had been admitted previously with a duodenal ulcer and the nurses indicated that on this occasion he had only been admitted to give his wife a rest because he pretended to be so helpless and was such a worrier about his bowels. He was very able to demand the nurses' attentions, although they observably turned deaf ears to his calls and avoided the vicinity of his bed as far as possible.

There were also three patients recovering from strokes who aroused the antipathy (somewhat guiltily expressed) of the majority of the nurses, including the sister. All three patients were aphasic or dysphasic, but two of them were able to make quite a noise when more than usually frustrated. One of them had been in the ward for over a year and attempts to transfer him to other accommodation had proved unsuccessful. There was a feeling on the part of all the staff that such patients should not be in an acute medical ward and they were placed in an area away from the other patients during the day. Attitudes towards their treatment and the consequent behaviour of these three patients differed noticeably in comparison with those of two similar patients in **Elm Ward.** There the ward sister particularly favoured the older dependent men and this seemed to be communicated to the nurses, several of whom counted one or other or both of the "stroke" patients among the ones they enjoyed caring for.

Summary

Patients the nurses least enjoyed caring for:
Grumbled and complained.
Communicated lack of enjoyment at being in hospital.
Implied that they were suffering more than was believed by the nurses.
Suffered from conditions the nurses felt could be better cared for in other wards or specialized hospitals.

Attitudes expressed by the nurses about patients they most enjoyed caring for

In the three medical wards, the most spontaneous and frequently given reasons for enjoyment in looking after patients related to the patients being fun or amusing, having a good sense of humour and being friendly and easy to get on with. In **Fir Ward** the majority of the nurses gave as their reason for enjoying caring for the most popular patient the fact that she was the most sensible. As one nurse said "Obviously you like the most sensible". It was the second most popular patient that the nurses found amusing and here the accent was placed on the fact that she was so entertaining and "you could not help laughing *at* her".

Sometimes a nurse would say that the person she most enjoyed looking after was a patient who did not rank high with any of the other nurses. In these instances the reason invariably given was that this was the patient they knew best, often explaining why this was so, such as the fact that they had "specialled" him when ill, or had accompanied him to a lengthy investigation; on two occasions the nurses had met these patients before in a different ward.

In two of the wards, the sisters indicated that among the patients they most enjoyed caring for were those they knew best because they had been in and out of the ward several times over a long period. In one instance a patient so mentioned was a man whom the rest of the nursing team said they did not enjoy looking after. Very few nurses spoke of the enjoyment they obtained from the actual nursing as a criterion for ranking the patients.

Summary

The majority of nurses included among the reasons given for choosing the patient for whom they most enjoyed caring, some reference to the patients being fun, having a good sense of humour, being easy to get on with and friendly.

Some individual preferences related to how well the nurses knew the patient.

Very few of the reasons given related to the nursing needs of the patients.

Attitudes expressed by the nurses about patients they least enjoyed caring for

Two main attitudes were expressed by the nurses about the patients they least enjoyed caring for, which linked with the two groups described under the behaviour of least liked patients. The first of these related mainly to the "grumblers" and "moaners" and the patients who demanded unnecessary attention, where the nurses described various feelings of frustration and impatience. For example, "He tries my patience to the limit. He is so pre-occupied with minor things and demanding attention when others need it", and "You can't get away from her". In exploring such sentiments further, the nurses indicated that the best way of dealing with people who demanded attention was to ignore them as far as possible and to show them that other patients needed the nurses' attention more than they did. Nobody could recall an actual incident of "being caught" by a patient and not being able to get away. It appeared that they were expressing a fear that this might happen rather than describing the discomfort of a remembered experience. If a nurse expressed this particular sentiment about a patient and later in the interview, when discussing what the nurse did during slack periods in the ward and the use of these for talking to or listening to the patients, the observer asked whether such a patient could provide a good excuse for stopping to talk for a while. This suggestion was mostly dismissed by indicating that if you gave in to such people you just stored up trouble by making them worse and no one would thank you for that.

The second attitude related to the patients whom the nurses felt did not need to be in hospital or whose condition did not warrant their being in that particular ward. In these instances the nurses expressed irritation that such patients wasted their time, to which sometimes an afterthought was added that perhaps they could not help it. On the whole they were dismissed as being nuisances or hypochondriacs, and in one instance as being psychopathic. When asked how they knew when a patient was genuinely suffering or "putting on" symptoms, the answers were that "you can just tell", or sometimes because the doctor or sister had told them. In one ward the sister was heard to explain during a reporting session that a patient's fainting attacks had been diagnosed as psychogenic; this did not mean that the nurses should ignore them, but just not make too much fuss about them, which showed that possibly she had an awareness of the nurses' natural inclinations. In another ward when the sister was talking about a patient admitted for investigation of abdominal pain who was known to have been treated previously for cancerphobia, she told the nurses not to take too much notice of him as he was just a hypochondriac with probably nothing the matter.

With regard to the patients whose condition the nurses felt was not suitable for their particular ward, the sentiments expressed implied a reluctance to provide the necessary care even though it was within the team's capabilities. For example, the three stroke patients in **Oak Ward** were grudged the amount of care they needed, albeit somewhat guiltily when expressed to the observer. In another ward a patient admitted in an unconscious state following a head injury elicited a lot of resentment about the amount of care he needed, whereas unconscious patients admitted to the same ward following cerebro-vascular accidents who needed the same amount of care and observation were given it unstintingly.

Sometimes the nurses' antipathy towards patients arose or coincided with the fact that they did not feel competent to provide the necessary care and this was particularly the case with patients diagnosed as being in need of psychiatric treatment. In all the wards extremely negative sentiments were expressed about such patients and sometimes the behaviour of the nurses seemed designed to exacerbate the patients' symptoms. The most extreme example of this occurred in **Fir Ward,** where an elderly woman was admitted with a diagnosis of agitated depression. The week before, a patient with senile dementia had been admitted who was considerably more noisy, restless and uncomprehending, but senile dementia was acceptable to the nursing staff and although this patient was not popular, she was fitted into the ward routine with the minimum of trouble. The woman with agitated depression was received and treated quite differently and the sister and permanent staff seemed to be glad when she proved "unmanageable" and was transferred to a psychiatric hospital. In one of the medical wards a patient admitted for investigation of headaches was diagnosed by the houseman as being an hysteric, and the nurses laughed at the accounts of him groaning whenever he was aware a member of staff was around. When a psychiatrist, who was asked to examine him, suggested he should have further investigations at another hospital as his symptoms were consistent with early cerebral tumour, he was totally disbelieved by doctors and nurses, but they arranged his transfer with such comments as "they are welcome to him" and "it won't take them long to see through him". Thus rejection or ridicule was usually the lot of such patients and the nurses either saw them as too "mad" for their care or else as playing up and not in need of hospitalization.

Summary

Frustration and impatience were expressed about patients who grumble, moan or demand attention, also irritation about patients considered to be wasting their time. Psychiatric patients were overtly rejected or ridiculed.

Use of Sanctions

Where rewards or deterrents are employed in a group situation they give some indication of which behaviours are approved and which disapproved, but it is an extremely elusive aspect to observe. When the nurses were asked how they might indicate approval to the patients they enjoyed caring for and disapproval to the patients they least enjoyed caring for they found it difficult to express. Several of them said they treated all the patients the same and three nurses ranked the patients only on the understanding that the order in which they placed the patients made no difference to the way in which they treated them.

When nurses did recognize that there was possibly some difference in their behaviour they were reluctant to verbalize what this might be, except in a very general way, such as "well I suppose I would be willing to put myself out more for someone like Mr. ——". These observations are, therefore, subjective interpretations of observed behaviour relating to those patients known to be more and less popular with the nurses.

Sanctioning behaviour could operate in several areas. Where the nurse came into contact with a patient because of carrying out a nursing task she could vary the way in which she approached a patient, the length of time she spent with him and the degree to which she personalized the interaction. The observer found these variations most noticeable when watching the ward sisters doing their daily round of the patients but they were also noticeable during temperature and medicine rounds and the serving of meals.

Other discriminatory behaviour was observed, particularly in relation to food. A patient might ask for a second piece of cake as the tea trolley returned past his bed and one might be given some, another refused and yet another given some but with a sarcastic remark. The same pattern was observed if a patient missed coffee through being out of the ward, with one person being allowed to get some for themselves, or having it fetched by a nurse, or being refused it. An unpopular patient who had been starved all day for tests to be carried out was given a plate of macaroni cheese for supper, which he did not fancy. He asked if there was any alternative and was told "No", but his neighbour asked another nurse for some ham and salad which was also one of the diet meals, instead of his macaroni, and when given some he exchanged his plate with that of the other patient.

Discrimination was especially observable in **Oak Ward** where rules for patients were most rigidly enforced, though some patients were allowed to smoke or have visitors out of hours without comment, while others were constantly chivvied and their relatives asked to leave.

The nurses seemed to think that ignoring patients was the most powerful deterrent to unacceptable behaviour and certainly some unpopular patients had requests ignored or forgotten. For example, when a staff nurse was doing a round of the patients a man asked if he could have his letters if the post had come as it was his birthday. She said she would look, then contacted the kitchen to order a special cake for his tea but appeared not to notice that the post was already on the desk. Over an hour and a half later the man asked a junior nurse and she went to ask the staff nurse who was sitting at the desk with the post in front of her. She picked the letters up, saying "I hope Mr. —— has got something as it's his birthday".

Apart from "forgettings" some other "ignoring behaviours" were probably not used as sanctions but were possibly due to the nurses' inexperience and lack of supervision, as when an elderly patient was given meat for lunch, which he was unable to cut up and when a patient who was supposed to be having complete rest had his lunch left on his locker and had to prop himself on his elbow in order to eat it. Similarly, patients described feeling upset when nurses chatted to each other, excluding them from the conversation, while carrying out care for them, but this seemed to be the practice of some nurses irrespective of whom they were caring for, rather than happening to just one or two patients.

A few positive rewards were seen to be given to patients as when the nurses clubbed together to buy a present for a girl who was having her birthday in hospital, and when the sister in one ward went to a great deal of trouble to arrange for a man to visit his crippled wife at home before he went to a convalescent home. Possibly the largest area of rewarding behaviour on the part of the nurses was the way in which they accepted favours from the patients. For example, laughing at jokes made by popular patients, accepting compliments and such things as sweets, fruit and newspapers from them, while refusing such offers from unpopular patients, unless they were given as a farewell present on their departure.

Summary
    Rewarding behaviour by the nurses:
        Willingness to give more time.
        Allowing a more personalized interaction.
        Willingness to accept gifts and favours.
        Allowing lapses in keeping the rules.
    Deterrent behaviour by the nurses:
        Ignoring the patients.
        Forgetting patients' requests.
        Refusing gifts and favours.
        Enforcing rules.
        Using sarcasm.

Observations of nurse/patient interaction in the wards
Patterns of interaction
    The most striking aspect of interaction patterns in all the wards was

that they were almost entirely task initiated. Nurses did not approach patients unless they were going to carry out some treatment or provide some service or unless they had some specific information they wanted to collect, and on the whole patients did not approach the nurses unless they had a specific need. There were some exceptions to this general pattern. In **Ash Ward** there was a junior pupil nurse who was able to make comments to the patients in general and if anyone responded she would carry on further conversation with them. If other nurses were not busy, such as when waiting for the meal-trolley to arrive for lunch, they would then gather round and join in.

In **Elm Ward** there was a Malaysian student nurse who was also State Enrolled, she would leave her colleagues when, in a slack period they had gathered in the sluice or treatment room, and approach elderly and lonely patients to get them talking and cheer them up.

Apart from these exceptions, it held true that on the whole when nursing tasks were completed the nurses removed themselves from the patient areas. This might have been because the observer was present, but remarks made by the patients indicated that this was a usual pattern. Thus one patient said "Sometimes there are so many nurses they are falling over each other to do things for you and then suddenly you can't get a nurse anyhow". Certainly, episodes were observed in each of the wards where one patient suddenly needed help and the other patients rang their bells or called and the observer was unable to find a nurse. After one of these episodes when a patient had fainted and seven minutes had elapsed before a nurse answered the bells, a patient said: "I dont' know where they get to—it's all right for me because I am independent, but I see the old ladies leaving their tea because they don't know whether they'll be able to get a bed-pan when they need one". This remark, made in a well-staffed ward, underlines another problem in nurse/patient interactions, which is the difficulty that some patients have in attracting a nurse's attention when there is one in the ward. Several of the nurses and some of the patients commented on the frustration and annoyance they felt when a nurse was interrupted in the middle of a task and it might be this that accounted for the singleness of purpose of some nurses while in the ward area that prevented them from hearing or seeing some patients' requests for help or attention. On a few occasions patients were purposely ignored or told curtly that they would have to wait; as these were the people who were classified as demanding or unpopular in other ways this very observable behaviour possibly helped to deter other patients from making requests.

One of the factors that distinguished popular patients was that they were able to attract the nurses' attention and initiate conversation with them and this was also observed by other patients who sometimes asked them to act as intermediaries in making their requests or voicing their complaints. If such a patient was ambulant, a bed-ridden patient might ask him for a drink of water or a urinal rather than "trouble" the nurses.

On the whole the patients seemed very well aware of each other's needs and were very alert to each other's condition when the nurses were not in sight. However, in all the medical wards there seemed to be a tacit understanding among the patients as to who they could do things for and who needed to have a nurse's attention. Thus in **Elm Ward** a patient recovering from a stroke, but still very helpless, was wheeled by the nurses into the sitting-room. Shortly after, the other patients left the sitting-room and returned to the ward, whereupon the man started calling for a nurse. The other patients had some chat and laughter about the nurses expecting him to stay in the sitting-room in the cold and eventually one of them went to see what he wanted. He asked to be wheeled back to the ward but was told that a nurse would have to do this. The ambulant patient returned to his fellows without getting a nurse and the calls started again until the ward maid went and wheeled him back to his bedside. An elderly man in the same ward, who was almost as helpless, was felt by the nurses not to be as incapacitated as he seemed. On some occasions the ambulant patients provided almost all his nursing care, such as helping him out of his chair and accompanying him to the lavatory while encouraging him to walk on his own, or cutting up his meat and making sure he had biscuits with a cup of tea when he hadn't eaten any lunch. It seemed as if the nurses were unaware of this, but on one occasion a nurse said "Mr. X will you try your charm on Pop? He won't take his tea for me". A comparable situation occurred in **Oak Ward** where there was another patient who was very helpless following a stroke, with hemiplegia and aphasia. He had been a very independent man and tried to continue that way in the ward. He was given a tripod walking aid but found it almost impossible to get out of his chair and would fall on the floor; as he had to climb four steps to reach the lavatory it was impossible for him to get there unless someone lifted his paralysed leg up each step. It was nearly always an ambulant patient who helped him up the steps and usually a patient who went to his aid when he fell. A nurse sometimes had to be collected to assist because he was so heavy but they did not go of their own volition if the patients got there to help first.

It was noticeable in all the wards that there were some patients who had practically no verbal contact with nurses or other patients for hours at a time. These would be patients who figured as neither popular nor unpopular and who were not acutely ill but were confined to bed. Routine tasks, such as temperature recording and serving of meals were carried out for them by nurse after nurse without a word being exchanged. For example, a patient in **Ash Ward** saw the nurse coming round to weigh everyone and when the scales were placed at the foot of her bed she got out of bed, stood on them, had her weight recorded and got back into bed without either of them saying a word. It is possible that such patients do not want to talk to anyone but it seems more likely that they could not take the initiative in starting conversation, since they talked with other patients when they were allowed up and could mix more freely, and did not rebuff any conversational openings offered to them.

Summary

Nurse/patient interactions were mainly task-initiated.

Nurses were not available in the patient areas when there were no tasks to be carried out.

Interactions with some patients were mainly non-verbal.

Joking, teasing and banter

Many of the interactions in the wards were conducted in a joking, teasing or bantering manner. There were a few patients and a few nurses who were particularly adept at initiating interactions of this sort, but other people would join in fairly readily.

Much of the conversation among groups of ambulant patients took the form of jocular banter and jocular grumbling. The subjects for the grumbling were for the main part of the food, the cold, noise and disturbed rest. There were innumerable examples in this area, fairly typical being exchanges such as:

"How's your lunch?"

"I never have gone much for seaweed." (Referring to the cabbage.)

"They should take some of the stalks out."

"Philip Harben wouldn't recognize it. They could make him feel useful here."

or:

"It's cold this morning."

"Trying to kill us off I expect—make room for the next blokes."

"They should issue us with fur coats, but they would have to be long ones."

Where the majority of patients were confined to bed there was noticeably less banter. Perhaps this was because it was impossible to obtain the necessary privacy. It also seemed as if bed patients made more overt complaints than ambulant patients and, while this was only an impression, it was true that practically all the patients whom the nurses stated they did not enjoy caring for because they grumbled and complained were confined to bed.

While the amount of bantering conversation between ambulant patients seemed fairly constant in the three medical wards, there was quite a difference in the amount of teasing and joking between patients and nurses, most being in **Elm Ward** and least in **Oak Ward**. The observer was convinced however that, since it occurred frequently, it was an important facet of communication. In the geriatric ward there was a little teasing and banter between some of the nurses and patients, but because of the nature of the patients' conditions and the fact that this ward had the largest number of foreign-speaking nurses there was only a small amount of lighthearted interchange.

Sometimes patients tried unsuccessfully to make jokes and usually they were the ones who were not very popular with the nurses. For instance, when a rather isolated patient had been taken for the first bath he had had for some time, he said to the nurse: "I feel a new man. That's my birthday bath" to which the nurse responded "Is it your birthday then?" "Yes" he said, "I only bath on my birthday!" This was said with laughter, but the nurse solemnly wished him "Many happy returns". Other patients got the point and laughed at the nurse, but she chided them for not greeting him also.

On some occasions remarks made by patients that were intended seriously were taken as jokes or teasing by the nurses. One example of this was an enquiry by a young lad with diabetes as to whether he should return the protamine zinc insulin which he had at home and no longer needed. He said "I've got fifteen bottles of 'protein' zinc insulin at home. Do you want them?" The nurse replied "Yes, I don't mind having some of *that*", and another patient joined in with "If it goes well with gin I'll have some too!" There was laughter and the nurse went away leaving the query unanswered. Another incident concerned a patient who had been given breakfast when booked for an I.V.P. which had then had to be postponed to the following day. At tea time he approached the nurses taking the trolley round and asked if he was allowed to have supper because of the test or should he have something extra to eat now. The nurses as a group responded teasingly, saying he shouldn't be worrying about supper when it was only tea time; as he was so lazy and lay on his bed all day he should be eating less, not more and no one actually answered his question.

It was observable that teasing and banter could be used in a rewarding way and in a deterrent way. A popular patient in one ward whose wife had sent him a large bunch of red roses on their wedding anniversary was teased in a way that enhanced the value of the roses both to him and to other patients who could see them. In the same ward there was a young Malaysian patient who was not very ill, not very cooperative and who tried to be too familiar with the nurses, demanding their attention. He constantly boasted about how much money he earned and two nurses colluded in saying that he would need a lot of money when he got the bill for his stay in hospital. He did not know whether to believe them or not and, when they went on kidding him, the librarian joined in agreeing with the nurses. Eventually, he started coughing and asked for some cough medicine. One nurse went away to fetch some linctus and came back with it, saying "It's only coloured water, but we'll make you pay for it". The nurses left the ward and after a while the patient approached another man to enquire about who did have to pay for treatment in the ward.

It was not uncommon for the patients to tease the nurses and many patients expressed appreciation of nurses who could take a joke. However, quite a number of nurses said that being teased by patients was one of the displeasures of nursing and, as one nurse said, the patients she did not enjoy caring for were the ones who teased her. It was possible for teasing to incapacitate a nurse, as when the patients in one ward were teasing a junior student nurse about which side of an extra bed to put a locker where there was very little space. Each side she put it they made up reasons why it should go on the other side, until she left it at the foot of the bed and went away. Eventually another nurse put it in place without a comment from anyone.

The patients' banter and teasing of the nurses could be rewarding or deterrent and, while comments about the nursing staff were usually sympathetic and favourable, if there were nurses or nursing situations that upset the patients they would come in for very ribald banter treatment. A nurse in one ward was so unpopular that the patients joined with other nurses when imitating and joking about her; in another ward a small group of patients tried to get the nurses to join in their complaining banter about the ward sister.

Summary

Joking, teasing and bantering interchange was common in the three medical wards.

Jocular grumbling, which occurred most among ambulant patients, appeared to limit formal complaining.

Teasing and banter were used in different ways with popular and less popular patients.

Nurses' attitudes to interaction with patients

When asked about the pleasures and displeasures in nursing, many of the nurses said that the things they enjoyed were working with people and the fact that nursing was never boring, and the things they disliked were being too busy, being interrupted while doing a task and not being treated with enough consideration by senior members of the nursing staff. When the observer tried to discover what constituted being "too busy" and when it had last occurred, it became apparent that this was an abstract fear rather than a reality frequently experienced; further discussion elicited the fact that all the nurses would rather be busy than not have enough to do. This held true in all the wards, but in **Fir Ward** the nurses felt they were kept busy most of the time, particularly the pupil nurses who were of the opinion that the work there was much too hard and physically exhausting and they thought they would become ill if they did not soon move to another ward.

In the medical wards the nurses described various feelings of distress and guilt they had experienced when there was not enough work to fill the time. They said it was possible to make some tasks, such as doing the medicine round, last a long time or else to find jobs to do outside the ward area. When asked how they viewed going into the ward and talking to or listening to a patient at such times, the concensus of opinion among the nurses was that your colleagues would consider you to be slacking if you did that and this made you feel guilty. On the whole they felt that the sisters in these wards would not mind, but in **Ash Ward** and **Oak Ward** they thought the sisters would check up extra well to make sure everything was done. If it was certain that all the necessary tasks had been done, it seemed to be more acceptable to read the patients notes than to go and talk to them.

The nurses were asked with whom, at the present time, they would have a conversation if they were sure that nobody would mind and, with one exception, they said it would be one of the patients they enjoyed looking after. The one exception was a nurse who said she would talk to someone who did not have any visitors, but when asked who was in this category at the moment, said there was no one, although this was the ward where one of the unpopular patients had complained of the embarrassment of not having any visitors.

On the whole, the impression gained from the nurses was that they enjoyed talking to and learning about patients as they carried out nursing tasks, but they did not feel there was any need for them to be more freely available for more of the patients and anyway there was no legitimate time for this. In **Ash Ward** to which student psychiatric nurses were seconded it was suggested by general student nurses that they talked to the patients too much, making them too dependent and unwilling to go home.

Summary

The nurses felt that they had enough conversation with patients while carrying out nursing tasks;

They felt guilty if they "chatted" to patients because their colleagues would think they were slacking;

They felt uncomfortable during slack periods in the wards but did not feel that having conversation with patients constituted "work" at such times.

If they stopped to talk to patients, nurses would choose the patients they most enjoyed caring for.

Patients' attitudes to interaction with nurses

Common to all the wards were comments from patients about how busy the nurses always were but how cheerful they managed to be in spite of this. If any omissions or mistakes were noticed, they were explained away and forgiven because the nurses had so much to do and so many things to think about. With this went a feeling that the nurses should not be bothered with trivial matters, and although some patients wished it was otherwise, it was a code that was strictly enforced by the patients among themselves, as well as being endorsed by the nurses. One patient who had been a nurse many years before was telling her neighbour about the discipline there used to be in the ward and how much easier it was when everyone knew "what was what". She said "Now the nurses are running all over the place and there is no peace, but they are not doing anything for you and you don't know where you are" and it was accepted by them both that there was nothing to be done about it. Referring to changes in the amount of discipline in the ward, another patient said, "It's the free and easy atmosphere that amazes me. You don't feel so in awe, but you need to know that things aren't going to slip—I don't think nurses notice things like they used to".

Several patients expressed bewilderment or anxiety about the number of nurses belonging to the ward and not being able to work out who was going to be there. One woman who had been in hospital many times previously explained to a recently admitted neighbour that, when she first comes in she picks a nurse she feels she can depend on and then when she is around asks her anything she needs, but patients with less experience of hospital had difficulty in determining who it was legitimate to interrupt in order to ask for something. In the two wards where there were ward clerks it was noticeable that many patients were able to approach them when they felt they should not bother the nurses. Sometimes the shyer patients would ask other patients to make requests for them or would seek reassurance that it was all right to ask.

Many of the patients implied that their own worries and needs were not serious enough for the nurses to be concerned about and, when talking among themselves, they quite often commented on the excellence of the care given to very ill patients and expressed confidence that as soon as anything was seriously wrong with anyone the nurses noticed and did something about it quickly and you could not really expect more of a hospital ward. There was, however, an undertone of regret that more time was not available for their concerns and occasional frustrated outbursts about being kept waiting or having nursing attention interrupted indicated a felt lack of attention.

Summary

The patients felt the nurses were too busy to be bothered with trivial matters.

Patients would welcome more opportunity to voice worries and needs, but felt this could detract from nursing care given to the seriously ill.

Summary of Part II

By a process of selective observation in four wards an attempt was made to explore and record the behaviour of nurses and patients as they interacted with each other. Popular and unpopualr patients were identified and special attention paid to any differences in the way the nurses behaved towards them.

Interviews with the nurses and talks with the patients explored some of the attitudes about roles in the ward situation and what constituted desirable and undesirable behaviour.

CHAPTER 11

Notes on the Theoretical Background to the Concepts of Small Groups, Group Norms and Role

This study relates to patients and nurses in the general ward situation and is based on the premise that, although the situation has certain unique features, the participants are subject to the laws that govern the behaviour of people in small social groups.

Originally, small social groups were called "primary groups" by Cooley (1909) and described as situations where all members could have a face to face relationship. Bales (1951) later used the term "small group" which he defined as being a group of any number of persons engaged in interaction with each other in a single face to face meeting or series of meetings where each member receives a distinct enough impression of every other one, and can either at the time or later give some reaction to each of them as an individual person.

Before examining small groups, consideration must be given to the individual as a social being. Born with the vital physical needs for air, food and water, warmth, rest and exercise and protection from dangers, the infant is utterly dependent on other people for the meeting of these needs and is, of necessity, involved in social interaction. To begin with the infant mainly takes, giving little other than "gratitude" and "co-operation" expressed by ceasing to cry when attention is given and by sleeping. However, if he is to continue to be given attention willingly, he must show approval and gratitude and, in order to learn how to do this he must first receive these things. It is through these exchanges that a person comes to have an awareness of his identity and the worth of his individuality.

As this learning takes place, the need for approval and affection becomes incorporated into the body's physiological need system, so that, when approval is not forthcoming anxiety is generated and experienced in the same way as when something like deprivation of food occurs. Thus a system of learned "social" or "emotional" needs comes to play a part in the motivation and behaviour of individuals.

A. H. Maslow (1954) has described human needs as a hierarchy developed in a specific order through childhood and adolescence; he suggests that, once developed, it is only when the needs of a lower order are met that the needs of the next impinge upon the individual, causing anxiety and distress and requiring to be met if contentment is to be achieved. He lists this hierarchy as follows:

1. Physiological needs, e.g. food, water.
2. Safety needs, e.g. protection from injury, pain.
3. Social needs, e.g. affection, approval, identification.
4. Esteem needs, e.g. prestige, self-respect, success.
5. Need for self-actualization.

Groups

In any society an individual needs the company and cooperation of other people, both for assistance in the tasks of living and in order to satisfy emotional needs. When people organize themselves into groups, both these factors play a part in keeping the group going, although some groups are formed mainly for the purpose of achieving a task, while others are formed mainly for companionship.

All groups are formed for some purpose but may vary greatly in the formality or otherwise of their organization, and in stability of membership. Where rules govern behaviour and members are appointed to designated positions, the group is referred to as being "formal", while a spontaneous gathering of people over a period of time is called an "informal" or "friendship" group. There can be varying gradations of formality in the organizations of groups and it is possible for informal groups to develop within a formal one.

Norms

Whether a group is formally or informally organized, the members will have an awareness of belonging and will have some place or position within the group that may relate to the task or the companionship area. In formal groups positions may be clearly defined and identifiable by means of uniforms or badges of office, while at the other extreme, positions in informal groups may only be defined at a subconscious level. Whichever the case, there will be consensus of opinion within the group about what behaviour is appropriate for the different "position incumbents" and for the membership as a whole. Various physical, social and moral frames of reference influence the prescriptions for acceptable and unacceptable behaviour in the group and these are termed "norms".

Homans (1950 and 1961) describes a norm as an idea in the minds of the members of a group, an idea that can be put in the form of a statement specifying what the members or other people should do, ought to do, are expected to do under given circumstances, and which elicits punishment in some form if behaviour departs too far from this ideal. Norms evolve from the tasks of the group and from the attitudes and

63

ideals of individual members, which in their turn have been inculcated in other group situations, such as the family, the school and the nation.

Role

When norms are applied to an individual by virtue of the position he holds in the group, this is referred to as his "role". "Role" is a complex concept and it is defined and classified in various ways, but the common denominator of most explanations is that it is the behaviour expected of an individual by virtue of his being the incumbent of a particular position in a social situation. The expected behaviour is sometimes referred to as the clusters of rights and obligations that relate to a particular social position. This description underlines the give and take of social interaction and, although it is recognized that participant members will differ in the nature and degree of the skills and abilities they can contribute, a competitive spirit is engendered in small groups. Such competition is for the approval, respect and recognition of individuality by the other members; it is achieved when the person fulfills his role prescription, abides by the norms and enhances the aims of the group.

The people who are accorded, or who earn the most respect and esteem have proportionally more influence over the other members and may be termed leaders. Klein (1956) observed that leaders arise in two main ways. The person who contributes most to the group's accomplishment of its task emerges as an "instrumental" leader and the person who contributes most to the companionship area emerges as an "expressive" leader. An instrumental leader is more likely to earn the respect of the group and the expressive leader to be best liked; if they co-exist there is always a potential status struggle between them unless the former is reconciled to sacrifice of popularity and the latter is reconciled to sacrifice of respect. Having been accorded influence as a leader, the individual can exercise this in ways ranging from the very autocratic to the very democratic. According to Klein, (1956) a person who is an appointed head in a formal group is sometimes referred to as a "formal" leader, but this person still has to earn respect or popularity with the members, in order to be able to influence them as an "actual" leader. These studies show that there are both pressures and needs for individuals to conform to group norms and, providing the norms are interpreted correctly and internalized, they will enact their roles according to expectations. Yet, in every act in a social situation the position of the individual in the group is at stake, in that an act may conform to the expectations of others and reinforce the present position, or it may deviate either in an acceptable or unacceptable way and lead to a rewarding or unrewarding change in position.

In spite of the pressures and rewards for conformity, it is recognized that there are individuals who, at any one time or frequently, do not wish or cannot conform to the norms of groups in which they find themselves and in consequence there has been a vast amount of study of what is termed "deviance". Deviance can arise for many reasons. An individual may not recognize the norms in operation, either through limited intelligence or other physical defect, or because not enough information is communicated; he may not be motivated to conform either because he is not in sympathy with the aims of the group or may not have learned how to earn esteem through cooperation; in the absence of adequate recognition of his worth while conforming in a group there may be more reward in having individuality recognized by not conforming. Whichever the case, the deviant member is likely to be unpopular with other members.

Many workers have attempted to devise scientific means of evaluating the extent to which members of a group accept or reject other members. Krech *et al.* (1962) *The Individual in Society*, state that Moreno, who coined the term "sociometry", was the first person to undertake such studies.

CHAPTER 12

Likes and Dislikes in Group Situations

It has been shown that people gather together in groups because they wish to achieve some aim that cannot be accomplished alone and that interaction with others comes to be, of itself, rewarding inasmuch as needs for approval and respect can be met by the other members. Thus in any group there will be two areas of motivation; to accomplish a task and to achieve a rewarding group solidarity; members will be evaluated for their contributions to these areas.

For individuals to become a group they must have opportunity to get to know each other and the interaction that occurs is both cause and effect of sentiments of liking that arise. Studies by Klein (1956) have shown that we like the people who have similar ideals to our own or who are what we would like to be, and we are willing to interact with them and show them esteem. On the other hand, the more people interact the more they come to find similarities and to like each other, though there must be some uniformity of ideals for this to occur.

As interaction proceeds a group ethos evolves, with behaviours and attitudes that are considered appropriate being defined either explicitly or implicitly, depending on whether the structure of the group is formal or informal. These behaviours and attitudes, termed norms, are compounded from the aims of the group and the ideals of the majority of the members. Because norms embody ideals that are, at least in part, the ideals of all the individuals, it is rewarding when others conform to them because this reaffirms their worth and demonstrates approval of them, therefore conformity is in its turn shown approval. On the other hand, if another member does not conform, this threatens the worth and validity of the norms and leads to feelings of insecurity and, therefore, the subscribers to the norms will bring pressures to bear to make the nonconformer come into line. Where nonconforming behaviour persists, the person comes to be regarded as a deviant and may well be referred to by a descriptive label that evokes a characteristic imagery and elicits responses such as contempt, suspicion, rejection or hatred.

In the nature of things, a group is more likely to be made up of members who get on well together, because the joint pressure that can be brought to bear on someone who does not fit in, will either change his overt behaviour and expressed attitudes (and may well modify and change his ideals) or will drive him from the group. This, however, only applies fully to informal groups where membership is voluntary and controlled by the participants. In formal groups, where membership is by appointment or assigned by circumstances, it may not be so easy to leave. Ideally in formal groups the ideals of the ascribed leader and all the members will concur and the group norms will come to incorporate these ideals. This will be evidenced by high morale and is most likely to occur where there is opportunity for all members to interact and make a contribution. In the opposite way, if this does not happen, there will be two main effects. First, there will be less motivation for members to reward and approve conforming behaviour, because it does not re-affirm their own ideals, and less motivation for individuals to conform to the ideals set by the group leader as conformity is less likely to be rewarded by others. Secondly, there will be a wider range of allowable behaviours making it more difficult for individuals to know where they stand in the evaluation system. This will be evidenced by low morale and is likely to lead to the formation of informal sub-groups where people of similar attitudes interact with each other as much as conditions will allow and establish their own norms within the formal group. While these informal groups are rewarding for the participating in-dividuals, they may or may not encourage them to enhance the aims or the tasks of the formal group. Whichever the case, other indivi-duals belonging to the formal group will try to obtain membership and when this is not forthcoming, they may well divert their energies to trying to disrupt the informal sub-group. If people's needs (for approval and self-respect in this instance) are not being met, they will experience frustration, but where they can see others having these same needs met, the frustration is greatly increased and jealousies arise that may well lead to feelings of dislike.

This indicates the ways in which evaluation systems evolve and result in people being liked or disliked in group situations where there is high or low morale. In practice the majority of groups do not fall distinctly into either category and thus both systems will operate to some extent.

Other factors influence liking and disliking in groups, which are extensions of the two systems already outlined. One of these is the phenomenon referred to as scapegoating. This is a situation that can occur in low morale groups when a leader or other dominant person forces members to contribute to the task area without there being sufficient rewards for so doing. This generates hostility among the members, but if the group is to continue and they are to remain within it, this hostility cannot be vented on the leader and is sometimes trans-ferred to another member or sub-group of members. This person, or persons, will be deemed unpopular, but because they serve a useful purpose, the hostility will not necessarily be expressed in such a way as to encourage them to leave the group and may well be tempered by such mechanisms as teasing or banter.

Another factor concerns people who are denied full social acceptance because they possess some sort of stigma. Because all individuals belong to many groups, they bring to any given situation attitudes and ideals that are the norms for them as members of a nation, of a family and of religious, political, work or leisure groups. Some of these norms will relate to expectations about people as fellow members of the human race and will form foundations for the development of concepts of normality and social acceptability that are termed stereotypes. If a person does not fall within the bounds of normality and is incongruous with a stereotype, his deviation is called a stigma. Goffman (1963) talks of stigma as "spoiled identity" and defines three different types: the physical deformities, such as blindness and paralysis; blemishes of character, such as weak will, dishonesty, mental disorder and homosexuality; and tribal stigmas of race, nation or religion. As with other deviation from norms, the person who is perceived as being abnormal will elicit feelings of discomfort in others. This may be experienced and reacted to in various ways. Basically, there will always be an impulse to reject the person, as there is with all persistent deviations from the norms and by its very nature stigma is seen as being immutable. However, many cultures teach their members to be accepting and kind to those with certain stigmas and then the person may be treated with sympathy and offered inclusion in groups; others however may still find it hard to be tolerant and so guilt may be added to their original discomfort which may make them reject the stigmatized person even more. Whether the stigmatized persons elicit sympathy or arouse guilt and hostility it is only rarely that their "difference" is completely discounted.

The term prejudice is used to described attitudes held about people who are not felt to be fully socially acceptable. Prejudice is described by Allport (1958) as a highly stereotyped emotionally charged attitude towards an object which is not easily changed by contrary information. Prejudices can be held about people and things and theoretically they can be favourable or unfavourable but usage tends to identify prejudice with unfavourable attitudes. Although prejudices are a function of individuals they are part of the attitudes and ideals that contribute to group norms, so that being more firmly entrenched they become part of the group's expression and identity. Where prejudices concern other people they are most strongly held about other individuals or groups who are seen to be threatening the group solidarity, or to be in competition for required resources and rewards and whose norms are suspected of being too different for them to be incorporated in the group (Krech and Crutchfield, 1962) and within a low morale formal group it is quite possible for prejudices to arise between sub-groups.

CHAPTER 13

Abstracts from the Literature on Popular and Unpopular Patients

1. *When a Student Dislikes a Patient:* Highley, B. L. & Norris, C. M., 1957. *Am. J. Nurs.*, No. 9, 1163–6.*
   Summarizes five major dislikes related to working with patients as described by American student nurses:
   1. Patients who feel bad and complain after everything has been done for them.
   2. Patients who are not clean.
   3. Patients who won't do what the nurse asks them to; won't cooperate; won't obey rules.
   4. Patients who can help themselves but insist on the nurse doing everything. Patients who cling to the nurse or "hang on to her coat tails".

2. *Who are "good" and "bad" Patients?:* Ritvo, M. M., 1963. *The Modern Hospital*, **100**, No. 6, 79–81.
   Some descriptive terms used by American student and graduate nurses to describe the "good" patient, obtained from 500 written questionnaires and over 1,000 informal interviews:

	%		%
Cooperative	83	Gets along with other patients	9
Appreciative	24	Pleasant personality	8
Cooperative and appreciative	16	Polite	8
Accepting own illness	13	Patient	8
Accepting prescribed treatment	11	Grateful	8
		Courageous	8
Understanding of illness	9	Sense of humour	7

   Responses to the definition of the "difficult" patient clearly pointed to the view that such a person had diametrically opposed characteristics to those of the "good" patient.

3. *Uncooperative Patients?:* Schwartz, D. R., 1958. *Am. J. Nurs.*, **58**, 75–77.
   Factors found to be common to 50 patients classified as "unco-

---

* For full references see Bibliography.

operative" by all categories of staff in an out-patient department in an American hospital.

1. All found it difficult to conform to the clinic routine.
2. All demanded attention in apparently excessive amounts.
3. All required immediate gratification of requests.
4. All responded immaturely to any pressures.
5. All possessed to a remarkable degree the ability to needle the professionally prepared people.

4. *Understanding the Nurse/Patient Relationship:* Ingles, T., 1961. *Nursing Outlook*, **9,** 698–700.

Sixty nurses in two American hospitals described the characteristics of "good" and "bad" patients.

"In rank order, the 'good' patient was judged because he possessed the following characteristics: non-complaining, non-demanding, co-operative with doctor's orders, appreciative of staff, helps self, physically and conversationally pleasing."

5. *The Problem Patient:* Harmuth, B., Lantz, U. & Oden, G., 1961. Unpublished paper. Rutgers, State University of New Jersey.

In an American hospital, 34 nurses designated 60 patients on wards selected for a study to determine the number of "problem patients" on those wards. Problem characteristics were ranked in eight categories, namely:

Communication	Overt emotional behaviour
Complaint	Physical care
Demand	Interaction
Interference from outside	Lack of cooperation

Within these categories 58 different characteristics were identified, of which the outstanding one was lack of cooperation.

6. *Be Kind to "Impossible" Patients—they're scared:* Viguers, R. T., 1959. *The Modern Hospital*, **92,** No. 1, p. 70.

There is a natural tendency to direct attention toward the "good" patient. The patient who is quiet, understanding, does as he is told and makes no unreasonable demands, is the one we are attracted to and spend most time with. However, it is the "impossible" patient who may need most attention and care. The easy thing is to try and avoid the patient who makes unreasonable demands, fails to follow instructions and seems unappreciative, whatever is done for him, but if we can understand some of the emotional aspects of being hospitalized, we can more readily give the difficult patient the added care and attention that he is asking for and needs.

7. *Social Science in Nursing: applications for the improvement of Nursing Care:* MacGregor, F. C., 1960. Russell Sage Foundation, N.Y.

Perhaps the most common label applied to patients by which they are identified and referred to by staff members is that of "good" or "bad".

These are terms within the hospital milieu that have specific meanings and are behaviourly defined. They are so usual that they amount to a stereotyped expectancy . . . . A good patient in this context is one who conforms to the medical regime . . . the prescribed treatment . . . nursing care and the rehabilitation programme and does so without questioning and without resistance. He does not make inconsiderate demands . . . . He is cooperative and reasonable, qualities usually equated with being "intelligent". He makes an effort to be a "good sport", tries to help himself and works at getting well. He shows appreciation for what is being done for him.

The "bad" patient is one who is difficult or uncooperative. He is likely to argue against or resist the required treatment. He questions everything that is done for him. Worse still, he may "know more" about his illness than the doctors and nurses. He is "emotional" and is likely to complain loudly or continually or both. He finds fault with the food, is inconsiderate . . . and is a constant "bell-ringer". He seldom shows any gratitude . . . .

8. *Care of the Adult Patient: Medical/Surgical Nursing:* Smith, D. W. & Gips, C. D., 1966.

Some patients continually complain about pains and aches or the service in the hospital. These patients are often disliked, particularly by the nursing staff . . . . The all too prevalent practice of calling patients who complain frequently (and some others) by such terms as "crocks" reveals lack of perception and understanding in the speaker.

9. *Professionalizer, Traditionalizer and Utilizer: an interpretive study of the work of the general duty nurse:* Habenstein, R. W. & Christ, E. A., 1955.

Just as any waiter can describe a "good" or "bad" customer, so quite naturally nurses develop and maintain images of the "good" and "bad" patient. . . . Patients who refuse to accept orders, who are "neurotic" or demanding are listed as problem patients. Treatment for this group generally becomes most perfunctory and impersonal.

10. *The Dynamic Nurse/Patient Relationship: function, process and principles:* Orlando, I. J., 1961.

. . . Behaviours are often termed "uncooperative", "unreasonable", "demanding" or "commanding". When the patient refuses to cooperate he prevents the nurse from carrying out activities which are designed for his well-being, and can prevent the nurse from liking him.

11. *Developing the Difficult Patient:* Peterson, D. I., 1967. *Am. J. Nurs.*, No. 3, p. 523.

"A difficult patient often is described as demanding, uncooperative, unresponsive to treatment, unappreciative or generally unlikeable. Actually a difficult patient is one whose needs are not met—emotional, physical, or both."

12. *A Critical Theory: The Nurse as a Fully Human Person:* Sarosi, G. M., 1968. *Nursing Forum*, vii, 4, p. 349.

"The characteristics of good and bad patients are not unfamiliar to most practising nurses. A 'good' patient has such attributes as emotional stability; he is cheerful, not overly anxious and keeps his feelings under control. He communicates easily with the nursing staff, is cooperative, is appreciative, conforms readily to hospital routine and policies, and is thoughtful of the busy nurse's point of view.

The 'bad' patient is emotionally unstable; he may be highly anxious, depressed and hostile. He may not communicate readily with nurses, he may challenge nursing actions or ask too many questions, he may be too independent. He is likely to be aggressive, impatient, unappreciative, unconforming to hospital routines and policies and unsympathetic to the nurses' point of view."

13. *Human Behaviour in Illness: psychology and interpersonal relationships:* Gillis, L. & Biesheuvel, S., 1962.

It is interesting to explore what kind of person and what sort of behaviour leads to a patient being termed "difficult" or "uncooperative" A common sort of behaviour . . . is that of the patient who is stubborn and will not easily accept the help being offered or given . . . shows a consistent lack of appreciation (may be due to language barrier, low I.Q. or hostility) . . . refuses to fall in with our own wishes and requirements.

Patients who behave thus usually have certain other features in common. They always seem to be wanting attention in excessive amounts and they demand immediate gratification. They tend to consider themselves invalids and even the way they ask for necessary things puts their attendants off . . . it will be seen that a patient is called uncooperative when he exhibits behaviour that is out of the ordinary run or with which our training and experience have not equipped us to deal. Such patients have the ability to needle the staff and make them respond abruptly or with irritation and anger . . . the total effect is to make those who have to deal with them feel ineffective.

Appendices

Tables showing Factors found to have no Significant Influence on the Popularity of Patients

TABLE 11

Classification of Patients by Popularity and Age

Marking	Class 1 ++		Class 2 +		Class 3 0		Class 4 —		Class 5 — —		Total
Age	Pts	%	Pts	%	Pts	%	Pts	%	Pts	%	
0–21	1	4	6	26	11	48	5	22	—	—	23
22–44	4	7	7	12	34	59	8	14	5	8	58
45–64	6	4	20	15	76	55	25	18	11	8	138
65 +	12	7	16	9·5	107	63	18	11	16	9·5	169
Totals	23	6	49	13	228	59	56	14	32	8	388 100%

These figures show no statistically significant difference between popularity and age.

TABLE 12

Classification of Patients by Popularity and Religious Affiliation

Marking	Class 1 ++		Class 2 +		Class 3 0		Class 4 −		Class 5 − −		Total
Religion	Pts	%	Pts	%	Pts	%	Pts	%	Pts	%	
C/E	17	6	35	13	158	61	35	13	18	7	263
R.C.	1	2	4	8	32	66	9	18	3	6	49
Non/Con	3	9	7	22	15	47	5	16	2	6	32
Jew	—	—	1	8	5	42	3	25	3	25	12
Other	1	9	—	—	5	45	3	27	2	18	11
None	1	6	2	12	8	50	1	6	4	26	16
Not Ascertained	—	—	—	—	5	100	—	—	—	—	5
Totals	23	6	49	13	228	59	56	14	32	8	388
											100%

These figures show no statistically significant difference between popularity and religious affiliation.

TABLE 13

Classification of Patients by Popularity and Social Class[1]

Marking	Class 1 ++		Class 2 +		Class 3 0		Class 4 −		Class 5 − −		Total
Social Class	Pts	%	Pts	%	Pts	%	Pts	%	Pts	%	
I	3	13	3	13	15	66	1	4	1	4	23
II	3	7	8	18	21	47	8	18	5	10	45
III	7	5	19	14	81	58	22	16	10	7	139
IV	7	10	8	12	42	61	7	10	5	7	69
V	1	3	6	16	25	69	2	6	2	6	36
Not Ascertained	2	3	5	7	44	57	16	21	9	12	76
Totals	23	6	49	13	228	59	56	14	32	8	388

These figures show no statistically significant difference between social class and popularity.

[1] The social class classification used is that of the Registrar General.

TABLE 14

Classification of Patients by Popularity and Type of Accommodation Prior to Present Admission

Type of Accommodation	Class 1 ++		Class 2 +		Class 3 0		Class 4 –		Class 5 – –		Total
	Pts	%	Pts	%	Pts	%	Pts	%	Pts	%	
With relative	15	5	34	12	160	62	42	15	16	6	267
With friend	3	14	2	9·5	13	62	1	5	2	9·5	21
Alone	5	5	13	13·5	51	53	13	13·5	14	15	96
Not Ascertained	—		—		4		—		—		4
Totals	23	6	49	13	228	59	56	14	32	8	388

These figures show no statistically significant difference between popularity and home living arrangements.

APPENDIX 2

Comments made by Nurses about Patients they most and least enjoyed caring for

(*a*) Distribution of the 120 *written* reasons given for enjoying looking after patients:

		Numbers	Percentage
Personality Factors			
Cheerful, happy bright		18	
Pleasant, nice		9	
Helpful		6	
Others		7	
	Total:	40	33
Communication Factors			
Grateful, appreciative		14	
Cooperative		9	
Uncomplaining		6	
Good sense of humour, jokes, livens things up, amusing		5	
Easy to talk to, friendly		4	
	Total:	38	32
Attitude Factors			
Understanding, thoughtful		8	
Willing to accept treatment		4	
Keen to get better		3	
Makes light of difficulties, optimistic		3	
Confident in staff		1	
	Total:	19	16
Nursing Factors			
Interesting to nurse		8	
Needs nursing		7	
Making good progress		5	
Ill		2	
In a long time		1	
	Total:	23	19

77

(*b*) Distribution of the 70 *written* reasons given for not enjoying looking after patients:

Personality Factors		Numbers	Percentage
Selfish, demanding, inconsiderate		11	
Unpleasant, etc., bad-tempered		7	
Unhelpful		5	
Not cheerful		2	
	Total:	25	36

Communication Factors		Numbers	Percentage
Uncooperative		8	
Difficult to talk to—get on with or get away from		8	
Ungrateful, never satisfied		6	
Complains, grumbles		5	
	Total:	27	38

Attitude Factors		Numbers	Percentage
Unwilling to accept treatment		2	
Does not want to go home		2	
Not as ill/helpless as he thinks		2	
Familiar		1	
	Total:	7	10

Nursing Factors		Numbers	Percentage
Not well known		4	
Does not need to be in hospital		1	
Needs psychiatric treatment		1	
Others		5	
	Total:	11	16

(*c*) Distribution of the 92 reasons given *verbally* for enjoying looking after patients:

Personality Factors		Numbers	Percentage
Cheerful, happy, bright		11	
Pleasant, nice		8	
Helpful		3	
Others		6	
	Total:	28	30

Communication Factors		Numbers	Percentage
Good sense of humour, jokes, livens things up, amusing		18	
Grateful, appreciative		8	
Cooperative		8	
Easy to talk to, friendly		4	
Uncomplaining		3	
	Total:	41	45

Attitude Factors			
Willing to accept treatment		4	
Keen to get better		3	
Makes light of difficulties		3	
Understanding		1	
Confident in staff		1	
	Total:	12	13

Nursing Factors			
Needs nursing		3	
In a long time		3	
Rational*		2	
Least trouble*		1	
Interesting to nurse		1	
Making good progress		1	
*Geriatric ward	Total:	11	12

(d) Distribution of the 71 reasons given *verbally* for not enjoying looking after patients:

Personality Factors		Numbers	Percentage
Unpleasant etc., bad tempered		11	
Selfish, inconsiderate, demanding		10	
Unhelpful		2	
Not cheerful		1	
	Total:	24	34

Communication Factors			
Complains, grumbles		10	
Uncooperative		6	
Ungrateful		3	
Difficult to talk to		3	
	Total:	22	31

Attitude Factors		Numbers	Percentage
Does not want to go home		2	
Questioning		2	
Unwilling to accept treatment		1	
	Total:	5	7

Other Factors		Numbers	Percentage
Needs psychiatric treatment		4	
Not getting better		2	
Not classified, e.g. vulgar 1 boring 1 heavy 1 fussy 1 etc.		14	
	Total:	20	28

APPENDIX 3

The Role Study

(a) Results of Using Role Definition Tool

Complete Agreement

1. It makes nursing much easier when patients are cheerful.....................
2. I always welcome patients' offers to help me if they are well enough to do so.....................
3. I think patients should help themselves as much as they can.....................
4. I like patients who make every effort to get better quickly.....................
5. I think patients like helping with jobs on the wards.....................

Majority Agreement

1. I do not like it when patients tell tales about each other.....................
2. Although I feel sorry for them I do not like it when patients are miserable.....................
3. I like it when patients express their gratitude to me.....................
4. I like patients to be tidy.....................
5. I think patients should be given instructions in a very simple form ....
6. I think patients should be willing to accept prescribed treatment.....................
7. I think it is important that patients should try to obey hospital rules ....
8. I think patients benefit if they cooperate with the nursing staff and do whatever they say.....................
9. I think patients who place themselves entirely in the doctors' and nurses' hands are better off than those who try to run their own treatment ....

10. It is important that patients should realize that they have to wait their turn for attention without making a fuss.....................
11. I think patients who are dirty upset the other people in the ward.....................
12. I think patients should always respect the authority of the medical team.....................
13. I admire patients who put on a brave face when they are in pain.....................
14. If they are well enough patients should offer to help with things like taking teas round.....................

Complete Disagreement
1. I want patients to tell me if other patients are breaking the rules.....................
2. I think patients should be allowed their own way while they are in hospital.....................

Majority Disagreement
1. It makes me feel annoyed when patients argue with me.....................
2. I find it displeasing when patients question the way in which I do things for them.....................
3. It makes life in the ward easier when patients are educated enough to take an intelligent interest in what is going on.....................
4. I expect patients to wait until I am not too busy before asking for things.....................
5. I find it rather difficult to cope with patients who insist on telling me about all their personal problems.....................
6. I like patients who are independent enough to refuse to take their drugs if they do not want them.....................
7. I get annoyed when patients make a lot of fuss when they are in pain
   ....
8. I find it embarrassing when patients give me presents while they are in hospital.....................

Divergent Opinion
1. I think patients should show gratitude for what they get in hospital
   ....
2. It is annoying when patients do not keep their beds and lockers tidy
   ....
3. I think patients should decline to have treatment they feel is not benefiting them.....................
4. I think patients should expect immediate attention whenever they think they need it.....................
5. I like patients who want my help with their particular personal problems
   ....
6. I think it is a good idea for patients to be allowed to do whatever they wish while in hospital, providing it does not interfere with their treatment.....................
7. It annoys me when patients make a fuss about taking their prescribed medication.....................
8. I think patients ought to be able to accept responsibility for reminding us about such things as urine saves and fluid balance charts.....................
9. I think nurses are justified in expecting patients to show appreciation for their care.....................
10. I think patients should show appreciation for their nursing care.....................

11. If patients feel neglected, I think they should demand attention..................
12. Patients who are clean and tidy are usually more popular than those who are not.....................
13. It is a pleasure to work with patients who take a real interest in their illness and treatment.....................
14. Although I should be sympathetic, I find patients who are very preoccupied with their illness rather trying.....................
15. Although it is often done, I do not think the patients should give the nurses presents.....................

	Totals
Complete agreement	5
Majority agreement	14
Complete disagreement	2
Majority disagreement	8
Divergent opinion	15
	—
Total number of statements:	44
	—

(b) Results of 12 Item Questionnaire

	Agree	Disagree	Don't Know
1. The more experience patients have had of hospitals, the easier they are to look after	6	30	2
2. Patients who can help around the ward are the most popular with nurses	11	21	6
3. Patients who have the most influence with the others are the easiest to deal with	6	22	10
4. Patients take a great deal for granted these days	20	12	6
5. Young patients are more nuisance than old ones	6	26	6
6. A tidy patient is a godsend	29	6	3
7. Men are easier to nurse than women	23	7	8
8. It is helpful from a nursing point of view when patients want to discuss their non-medical personal problems	27	4	7
9. Patients who express appreciation are more likely to get attention than others	16	21	1
10. Patients need to be adaptable to get on well in hospital	34	2	2
11. Well educated patients are more satisfying to nurse than others	8	25	5
12. A cooperative patient is likely to get well quicker than an uncooperative one	33	2	3
Totals:	219	178	59

APPENDIX 4

Data Collecting Schedules

1. Rating Chart

Rating chart

Hospital				1
Ward				2
Nurse				3

Below is a list of the patients in your ward.

Would you please rate them in the following way:-

I enjoy looking after this patient very much	– A
I quite enjoy looking after this patient	– B
I do not enjoy looking after this patient very much	– C
I do not enjoy looking after this patient	– D

If you are unable to rate a patient would you give the reason why.

(For example:– I don't know this patient yet.
I don't have any definite opinion.
.... any other reason.)

What you put on this form will be completely confidential, and the investigator will not study the ratings until she has left.

	NAME	ABC or D	or REASON FOR NOT RATING
1			
2			
3			
4			
5			
6			
7			
8			
9			
10			
11			
12			
13			
14			
15			
16			
17			
18			
19			
20			
21			
22			
23			
24			
25			
26			
27			
28			
29			
30			

2. Classification of Patients

1 □ 2 □	Hospital	1 2
3 □ 4 □	Ward	3 4
5 □ 6 □ 7 □	Patient	5 6 7
8 i ii	Sex: Male i Female ii	8
9 i ii iii iv v	Age: -15 i 16-21 ii 22-44 iii 45-64 iv 65+ v	9.
10 i ii iii iv v vi	Religion: C/E i R.C. ii Non.Con. iii Jew iv Other v None vi	10
11 i ii iii iv v vi vii viii	Length of stay to end of observation 11 period Less than one week i One week and less than one month ii One month and less than three months iii Three months and less than one year iv One year and over v Information not accurate vi Information not obtained vii None viii	11
12 i ii iii iv v vi vii viii	Length of previous admission to this hospital Code as above i ii iii iv v vi vii viii	12
13 i ii iii iv v vi vii viii	Length of admissions to other hospitals Code as above i ii iii iv v vi vii viii	13
14 i ii iii iv v vi vii viii ix	Country of origin England i Wales ii Scotland iii N. Ireland iv Eire v West Indies vi Africa vii Asia viii Other ix	14
15 i ii iii iv	Language Specify if native language is other than English .... Length of time English has been used .... Length of residence in England .... English comprehension rating Good i Fair ii Poor iii None iv	15

Contd.......

		Patients
6 i ii iii iv v vi vii viii ix x xi xii xiii xiv xv xvi	<u>Diagnosis</u>	16
7 i ii iii iv v vi	<u>Defects:</u> None i Disfigurement ii Obesity iii Deafness iv Aphasia v Other vi	17
8 i ii iii iv v vi vii viii	<u>Nursing Factors</u> None i Unconscious ii Semi-conscious iii Confused iv Incontinent v Catheterised vi Unable to get out of bed alone vii Needs feeding viii	18
19 i ii iii iv v	<u>Occupation</u> Subject Husband Father R.G. Classification i ii iii iv v	19
20 i ii iii	<u>Marital Status</u> Married i Single ii Widowed iii	20
21 i ii iii	<u>Accommodation</u> Living with relative i Living with friend ii Living alone iii	21
22 i ii iii	<u>Participation</u> + + i + ii Limited or nil iii	22

3. Nursing Staff Questionnaire

1. 2. ☐ ☐	Hospital	1 2
3. 4. ☐ ☐	Ward	3 4
5. 6. 7. ☐ ☐ ☐	Nurse	5 6
8 i ii	Sex: Male i Female ii	8
9 i ii iii	Age: Under 30 i 30-44 ii 45+ iii	9
10 i ii iii iv v vi	Religion: C/E i R.C. ii Non.Con. iii Jew iv Other v None vi	10
11 i ii iii iv v vi	Grade: Sister/C/N i Staff Nurse ii Enrolled nurse iii Student iv Pupil v Auxiliary vi	11
12 i ii iii iv v	Length of time in active nursing Up to three months i 3 months up to one year ii 1 year up to 3 years iii 3 years up to 5 years iv Over 5 years v	12
13 i ii iii iv v	Length of time at this hospital Code as above i ii iii iv v	13
14 i ii iii iv v vi vii viii ix	Country of origin England i Wales ii Scotland iii N. Ireland iv Eire v West Indies vi Africa vii Asia viii Other ix	14
15 i ii iii	Length of residence in G.B. .... Native language .... English Good i Fair ii Poor iii	15
16 i ii iii iv v	Age on leaving school 14 or less i 15 ii 16 iii 17 iv 18+ v	16
17 i ii iii iv v	Educational qualifications None i 1-3 'O' Levels ii 4 or more 'O' Levels iii 1 or more 'A' Levels iv Other v	17
18 i ii iii iv v vi vii	Professional qualifications S.R.N. i R.M.N. ii R.S.C.N. iii S.C.M. iv S.E.N. v Other ...... vi None vii	18
19 i ii iii iv v	Father's occupation	19

86

List of Statements about Patients

Below is a list of statements about patients.

Please would you indicate how you feel about these statements by ticking the appropriate column.

	Agree	Dis-Agree	Don't Know
1. The more experience that patients have had of hospitals the easier they are to look after.			
2. Patients who can help around the ward are the most popular with nurses.			
3. Patients who have the most influence with the others are the easiest to deal with.			
4. Patients take a great deal for granted these days.			
5. Young patients are more nuisance than old ones.			
6. A tidy patient is a godsend.			
7. Men are easier to nurse than women.			
8. It is helpful from a nursing point of view when patients want to discuss their non-medical personal problems.			
9. Patients who express appreciation are more likely to get attention than others.			
10. Patients need to be adaptable to get on well in hospital.			
11. Well educated patients are more satisfying to nurse than others.			
12. A co-operative patient is likely to get well quicker than an unco-operative one.			

Bibliography

ALLPORT, G. W. (1958). *The Nature of Prejudice*. Doubleday Anchor Books, N.Y.

BALES, R. F. (1951). *Interaction Process Analysis*. Addison Wesley Press Inc., Cambridge, Mass.

BANTON, M. (1968). *Roles. An Introduction to the Study of Social Relations.* Tavistock Publications.

BIDDLE, B. J., & THOMAS, E. J. (1966). *Role Theory*. J. Wiley & Sons, N.Y.

CAIN, M. E. (1968). Suggested developments for Role and Reference Group Analysis. *British Journal of Sociology*, 19, No. 2, p. 191–205.

COHEN, A. K. (1966). *Deviance and Control*. Prentice-Hall Inc., N.Y.

COOLEY, C. H. (1909). *Social Organization, A Study of the Larger Mind.* Scribners, N.Y. (Quoted by T. M. Mills).

DAVIS, K. (1949). *Human Society*, 2nd edition. Macmillan, N.Y.

ETZIONI, A. (1968). Basic Human Needs, Alienation and Inauthenticity. *American Sociological Review*, **33**, 6, 870.

FESTINGER, L. (1954). A Theory of Social Comparison Processes. *Human Relations*, VII, (Quoted by J. Klein).

GILLIS, L. & BIESHEUVEL, S. (1962). *Human Behaviour in Illness; psychology and interpersonal relationships.* Faber.

GLASER, B. G. & STRAUSS, A. L. (1965). *Awareness of Dying*. Weidenfeld & Nicolson.

GLASER, B. G. & STRAUSS, A. L. (1968). *The Discovery of Grounded Theory.* Weidenfeld & Nicolson.

GOFFMAN, E. (1956). *The Presentation of Self in Everyday Life.* University of Edinburgh.

GOFFMAN, E. (1963). *Stigma; Notes on the Management of Spoiled Identity.* Prentice-Hall Inc., N.Y.

GROSS, N., MASON, W. S. & McEACHERN, A. W. (1958). *Explorations in Role Analysis.* John Wiles & Sons Inc., N.Y.

HABENSTEIN, R. W. & CHRIST, E. A. (1955). *Professionalizer, Traditionalizer & Utilizer. An Interpretive Study of the Work of the General Duty Nurse.* Univ. of Missouri, Columbia, Mo.

HARMUTH, B., LANTZ, U. & ODEN, G. (1961). *The Problem Patient.* Unpublished paper. Rutgers, State Univ. of New Jersey.

HIGHLEY, B. L. & NORRIS, C. M. (1957). When a Student Dislikes a Patient. *American Journal of Nursing*, **9**, 1163.

HOMANS, G. C. (1951). *The Human Group.* Routledge & Kegan Paul.

HOMANS, G. C. (1961). *Social Behaviour: its elementary forms.* Routledge & Kegan Paul.

INGLES, T. (1961). Understanding the Nurse-Patient Relationship. *Nursing Outlook*, Vol. 9, No. 11, p. 698.

KLEIN, J. (1956). *The Study of Groups*. Routledge & Kegan Paul.

KRECH, D., CRUTCHFIELD, R. S. & BALLACHEY, E. L. (1962). *The Individual in Society: a textbook of Social Psychology*. McGraw Hill.

LAMBERT, W. W. & LAMBERT, W. E. (1964). *Social Psychology*. Prentice Hall, New Jersey.

LINTON, R. (1936). *The Study of Man*. Appleton Century, N.Y.

LINTON, R. (1947). *The Cultural Background of Personality*. Routledge & Kegan Paul.

MACGREGOR, F. C. (1960). *Social Science in Nursing: Application for the Improvement of Patient Care*. Russell Sage Foundation, N.Y.

MADGE, J. (1963). *Origin of Scientific Sociology*. Tavistock Publications.

MASLOW, A. H. (1970). *Motivation and Personality*, 2nd edition. Harper & Row, N.Y.

MERTON, R. K. (1957). *Social Theory and Social Structure*, 9th edition. The Free Press, Glencoe, N.Y.

MORENO, J. L. (see Krech, D., Crutchfield, R. S. & Ballachey, E. L., ref. p. 390).

MILLS, T. M. (1967). *The Sociology of Small Groups*. Prentice-Hall Inc., N.Y.

NADEL, S. F. (1951). *The Foundations of Social Anthropology*. Routledge & Kegan Paul.

ORLANDO, I. J. (1961). *The Dynamic Nurse-Patient Relationship: Function, Process and Principles*. Putnam, N.Y.

PARSONS, TALCOTT (1964). *Social Structure and Personality*. The Free Press of Glencoe, N.Y.

PETERSON, D. I. (1967). Developing the Difficult Patient. *American Journal of Nursing*, p. 522.

RITVO, M. M. (1963). Who are good and bad patients? *Modern Hospital*, **100**, 6, 79.

SAROSI, G. M. (1968). A Critical Theory: The Nurse as a fully Human Person. *Nursing Forum*, **VII**, 4, 349.

SCHWARTZ, D. R. (1958). Unco-operative Patients? *Am. J. Nurs.*, 75.

SMITH, D. W. & GIPS, C. D. (1966). *Care of the Adult Patient: Medical-Surgical Nursing*, 2nd Edition. Lippincott, Philadelphia.

SNYGG, D. & COOMBS, C. H. (1949). *Individual Behaviour*. Harper, N.Y.

SOUTHALL, A. An Operational Theory of Role. *Human Relations*, Vol. XII. (Quoted by Banton.)

SPROTT, W. J. H. (1958). *Human Groups: a Study of how Men and Women behave in the family, the village, the crowd and many other forms of association*. Penguin Books.

VIGUERS, R. T. (1959). Be kind to impossible patients—they're scared. *The Modern Hospital*, **92**, 1, 70.